Perfume:

Homemade Ecstasy

William Ziegler

CONTENTS

ACKNOWLEDGMENTS

First and foremost I would like to thank my sister Kat Gasior for help editing my work and support she gave. Mary Michelle Sanchez for helping find myself when I was lost and helping me to believe in myself. My children for making me be stronger than I ever was. Meredith Herman for spawning my interest in fragrance industry.

Prelude

I believe wearing perfumes and colognes are a way that people around the world treat themselves to a little bit of ecstasy. Why do women love perfume so much? Some researchers believe that a woman's reason for loving perfume is because of the pheromones their bodies produce. Certain scents and perfumes can trigger the increase of how much pheromone a woman's body will produce. Most women in the world will purchase perfume at least once or twice each year. Perfumes are liked by women because of the attention they get from a member of the opposite sex or even from another woman. Many women will tell you that the reason they purchase a particular perfume for themselves is that perfume makes them smell great and they seem to feel better about them. It also makes them feel a little bit more feminine. In some women perfume raises their confidence and in turn makes them feel more attractive.

In this book, you will be looking at ways of how to make your own perfume. You will be able to learn how to produce scents. Plus understand the general understanding of how to make new ones.

CHAPTER 1
THE BRIEF HISTORY OF PERFUME

The use of aromas, fragrances, and scents has been used for many centuries. Over the years, evidence has been found through archeological findings, as well as texts written by our ancestors, that has shown just how aromas were being used. In the very early civilizations, scented flowers and herbs were used by people to worship the Gods, and when burned, some of these plants would release strong aromas. Such scented fires became part of many religious rituals. In fact, you will find that many religions still use scented fires today.

Both the Assyrians and Egyptians used scented oils. The demand for the raw materials needed to produce both fragrances and remedies led to the discovering of new ways of extracting scents from the plants they used. Such techniques as pressing, decoction, pulverization and maceration were developed and mastered by both the Assyrian's and the Egyptians. They even made attempts at trying to produce essential oils by distillation.

The Bible describes a sacred perfume consisting of liquid myrrh, fragrant cinnamon, fragrant cane, and cassia. Its use was forbidden, except by the priests. The woman wore perfume to present their beauty.

The Persians used scents and perfumes as a sign of wealth or even rank. The Persians were famous for the red rose scent. They also enjoyed jasmine, lilacs and violets. The Persian Muslim doctor and chemist Avicenna introduced the process of extracting oils from flowers by means of distillation

The use of perfumes spread to Greece. Perfumes were used in religious ceremonies, and also for personal purposes as well. According to Greek mythology, the gods were responsible of teaching the use of perfumes to the men and to the women.

The Romans began to use fragrances even more lavishly. There are many manuscripts around describing the herbs which they brought from all over the world to produce the fragrances they used. The Romans used scents in religious ceremonies to celebrate the goddess of Flora.

During the Middle-aged, perfumes again were being used in churches in Europe for religious ceremonies. Aromatic Baths were taken to cover the stench caused by the many diseases which abounded at this time.

The Orient was reestablished at the beginning of the 13th Century, exotic flowers, herbs and spices became more readily available around Europe. Venice quickly became the center of the perfume trade. It was not long before perfumery soon spread to other European countries. The perfume trade then developed even further, as those returning from the crusades reintroduced perfume for personal use. In France the perfume industry flourished. France emerged as the European Center for perfumes.

The late 18th Century, the synthetic material fragrance was being produced, and this was the beginning of perfumery in the modern age. Thus with the introduction of synthetics, perfumes would no longer be exclusively used by the rich and famous. The synthetics were now being used to produce perfumes; perfumes could now be made on a much larger scale, although naturals were still also being used to help soften the synthetics. Today, natural products still remain a very important part of the production of perfumes in modern formulations. The Eau de Cologne was invented at this time and was nicknamed Water from Cologne. Jean Marie Farina invented it in Cologne, Germany. Eau de Cologne was a big success in all of Europe.

CHAPTER 2
WHAT CAN YOU USE TO MAKE PERFUME?

Most perfume that you purchase or make yourself is a chemical compound made from aroma blends; fixatives, fragrant oils and solvents. These all produce pleasant or attractive smell. Primarily women use perfume in order to smell nice if they are attending a special event, or to help attract another person.

The composition of any perfume starts with base perfume oils, which are natural, animal or synthetic, and are then watered down with a solvent to make them light and applicable. Unfortunately, perfume oils in either pure or undiluted form, can cause damage to skin, or an allergic reaction, so the adding of solvent is necessary to make them less potent. The most prevalent solvent used in the manufacturing of perfumes is Ethanol.

Plants are the oldest source for obtaining fragrant oil compounds from, and the parts used the most are the flowers and blossoms. There are other plant parts that can also be considered for use in perfume making bulbs, leaves, fruit, roots, rhizomes, seeds, wood, twigs, bark and lichens.

Perfumes that have been made using animal sources, they are normally made from Musk. Musk is obtained from either the Asian Musk Deer or Civets (known as Civet Musk), as well as Ambergris (a fatty compound). Some perfume makers may also use either Castoreum or Honeycomb in the production of their perfumes.

As for synthetic source perfumes, these are produced through organic synthesis of multiple chemical compounds, and such things as Calone, Linalool, Coumarin and Terpenes are used to make synthetic fragrant oils. By using synthetic products in perfume making, you can produce smells which are both unnatural, and which may not even exist in nature, have become very valuable element in the making of perfumes.

Perfumes are made in order to attract the customer via the olfactory system (sense of smell) in order to persuade people to buy the perfumes or perfume laced products that they are producing. A perfume composition will either be used to augment other products, or patented and sold as a perfume after it has been allowed to age for one year.

Fragrance compounds will, after time, begin to deteriorate and lose strength if stored incorrectly. It is important when thinking about making your own perfume, that you store them in tightly sealed containers, and keep them out of light and away from heat, as well as away from oxygen and other organic substances. If you want to get the best results possible the containers should be stored in a fridge at a temperature of between 3* to7* degrees Celsius, that is 37* to 45* Fahrenheit.

Today more than ever, perfume is popular around the world because both its use and application continues to grow.

CHAPTER 3
THINGS TO THINK ABOUT BEFORE STARTING

In this chapter of the book we will look at a few simple ways in which you can make your own perfume for next to nothing.

Research has shown that you can actually make a 100 bottles of perfume for less than $300, and then, if you want, sell them for up to $50 each.

Certainly some of the most profitable perfumes that are now available are ones which have not cost much to produce.

Previously when people were looking to produce their own perfume it was very difficult to find the ingredients, along with the packaging (bottles, spray nozzles etc.). But this has all now changed due to the internet and being able to order things online. Today you will find that you can obtain the ingredients you need at a reasonable price, and have the order sent directly to your home address.

However, there are some things which you will need to remember before you commence making your own perfume.

1.   You first need to think of a name for your perfume. You should use something catchy so people will remember it.

2.   Now you have the name, you need to design a label. The label being small simple artwork would be best.

3.   Next you need to look at what kinds of ingredients you will require, and make a list.

4.   Search for the best types of bottles, lids and pumps that you will need to put your perfume into you want your perfume to look good.

5.   Next you will need to spend a couple of days choosing your fragrances. It is important that you carry out as much research as possible on any other ingredients that you should use.

6.   When preparing the ingredients, it is important that you are in a sterile environment. Sterilize all equipment before pouring the perfume into the bottles you have chosen and bought.

7.   Finally, look at a way in which you can present the finished product to customers. Displaying in a box or a small gift basket.

You can see producing your own perfume is a simple process and if it is something you have always considered doing   then   why   not   give   it   a   go.

CHAPTER 4
HOW TO START MAKING YOUR OWN PERFUME

Whether you have decided to make perfume for yourself or for family use, or even as a gift for a loved one or friend, perfume is in fact something you can easily do by yourself or with others. Certainly producing your own perfume is not only a great way of learning a new skill, but it may also boost your confidence, and most importantly, you will have fun when doing it.

If you carry out a search on the internet on "making perfume or perfume recipes", you will soon find there is a wealth of knowledge out there on the many ways and different recipes to make it. The most important thing you should think about before making any decisions, is what sort of perfumes it is you would like as your finished product to be.

You will need to consider what sort of perfume it is you would like to make? Would it be an eau de cologne, perfume concentrate or even an aftershave? You will also need to decide what it should smell like? Do you want it to be soft or strong, sweet or manly or unisex? Does it have to be long lasting?

Now that you have made a decision by answering the questions .You need to start making a list of the ingredients that you need. When making the list, you should think about the characteristics of the various ingredients that you want to include in your recipe. However, if you already have a recipe that you would like to use, it may mean you do not need to bother experimenting with the ingredients you have. You may want to adjust the quantities of the ingredients you are using in order to make the perfume more personalized. If you do not have your list of ingredients already prepared, then there are a couple things that you should know prior to making your list.

When making perfume it is important that you experiment as much as you can. It should be remembered that perfume making is an art, and imagination and a great sense of smell will help you to overcome any lack of knowledge or experience that you have.

The next most important thing in relation to perfume making is that there are 3 key ingredients you will need to produce perfume:

1.   Essential Oils
Essential Oils have been extracted from various plants. They can be organic or non-organic .When Essentials Oils combined, they will give the smell of the perfume you are trying to produce.
2.   Alcohol
3.   Pure Water

There is 3 different Types of oils used in perfumes will ultimately influence the smell of perfume over time.

1.   The Base Oil (Base Notes) – This will produce the scent that stays longest on the skin and for this reason it is usually added to the mixture first.

2.   The Middle Oil (Middle Notes also called Hearth Note) – This also influences the smell of the perfume for quite some time, but not as long as the base notes does.

3.   The Top Oils (Top Notes) – This is added to the mixture after the middle notes, and may then be followed by some other substance which will help to bridge the scents together.

It is very important that when you are making perfume, you mix the extracts in the above order, and that you use enough of each type, most of the time equal amounts in order to produce the right sort of perfume.

Below are provided a list of oils that you can obtain and which will help you to produce the perfume of your dreams.

1.   Base Notes – Sandalwood, Vanilla, Cinnamon, Mosses, Lichens, Ferns, Amber, Ambergris, Opoponax, Balsam Peru, Oakmoss, Cedarwood, Clove, Cassia, Frankincense, Jasmine, Myrrh, Neroli, Rose, Rosewood, Valerian, and Ylang-ylang

2.   Middle Notes – Lemon Grass, Geranium, Neroli, Bay, Black Pepper, Cardamom, Chamomile, Cypress, Fennel, Geranium, Ho Leaf, Ho Wood, Hyssop, Juniper, Lavender, Marjoram, Melissa, Myrtle, Nutmeg, Palma Rosa, Pine, Rosemary, Spikenard, Yarrow

3.　　Top Notes – Orchid, Rose, Bergamot, Lavender, Lemon, LimeBasil, Bergamont, Cajuput, Cinnamon, Clary Sage, Coriander, Eucalyptus, Grapefruit Hyssop, Lemongrass, Lime, Mandarin Neroli, Tangerine Nerloi, Verbena, Niaouli, Orange, Peppermint, Petitgrain, Ravensara, Sage, Spearmint, Tagetes, Tangerine, Tea Tree, Tyme.

The list above is just a faction of the possibly you can have. A lot of the Notes can move up from Base Note to Middle Note or Middle Note to Top Note.

CHAPTER 5
SETTING UP AND EQUIPMENT

Now that you have made a decision to produce your own perfume, whether to earn an extra income or just as a hobby, you will need to start looking for places where you can get your supplies from. So in this chapter of the book we will look at ways of getting the necessary supplies in order for you to make your own perfume.

1.   First, you will need to choose a formulation or perfume recipe. The reasons perfumes differ is down to the formulation or recipe that has been used, and in order for you to produce a perfume that people will like, it is necessary to choose a good recipe or formulation.

It is very important that you decide what kind of perfume it is you want to make, and then read through the description of a particular recipe, to see if it will produce the desired result you are looking for.

2.   Next, you will need to look at essential and fragrance oils that are available. These are one of the major ingredients in the making of perfumes, it is important that you choose ones which are of a good quality. The better quality oils you use the better quality your finished product will be.

The oils used will establish the perfume's inherent attributes, like mood, quality and character. What you should remember, however, is that essential oils are much more expensive than fragrance oils. When first starting out, it may be wise to just use fragrance oils only to save on money until you've become more skilled.

3.   Any perfume made today is not made with fragrance or essential oils alone, and alcohol is also used as the primary solvent (helps to reduce the strength of the oils).

4.   When making any homemade perfume, it is important that you use the right materials for not just measuring, but for handling, mixing and storing the finished product in.

5.   You should use measuring devices that allow you to exactly measure out the amounts of oils and solvents required. If you do not, the perfume you make may not be what you wanted. It is best if you use measuring devices made from glass so that you can see what is inside and when handling any formulas then use a funnel with a narrow long neck.

6.   Fixatives are used with the other ingredients in order to lower the rate of evaporation of the fragrance or essential oils. The reason why a perfume may lose its fragrance faster than normal is because only a little amount of fixative was used when preparing the perfume

7.   It is important that you learn about, and understand, the health risks which are associated with essential and fragrance oils. There may be some formulations or recipes which could cause health problems if the oils included in them are used incorrectly.

Now that you know what supplies you need to use to make perfume, you need to know where to get them. You may be able to get them from a shop in your area. I would suggest craft stores. You could also go online, as there are plenty of places which sell perfume kits. Simply do a search for "perfume kits", and you will soon see what is available. You can also look for craft stores

CHAPTER 6
SIMPLE PERFUMES AT HOME

To recap the 3 main ingredients which you will need are:

1. Essential Oils
2. Distilled Water
3. Alcohol

Many of these items can be either obtained from a store that specializes in such ingredients, or over the internet. You will also need a large saucepan, large bowl spoon and some measuring cups or jugs to make perfume at home.

Here are a few easy recipes that you should be able to produce at home

1. **Basic Recipe**
All you need for this recipe is some water and chopped flower blossoms. You can use lilac or lavender if blossoms are unavailable.

Place the flower blossoms in a bowl, add the water and then cover them and leave them overnight. The next day, the solution can be put into small bottles and sprayed either into the air or on to your skin.

2. **Amaze Night**

For this, you will need some distilled water, vodka, hypericum perforatum, cypress and rosemary. They are all are essential oils. They should then be mixed together and stored overnight.

a. 2 cups distilled water
b. 3 tablespoons vodka
c. 5 drops hypericum perforatum which is also called St.John's Wort
d. 10 drops cypress
e. 10 drops rosemary

After a period of 12 hours or more, the solution produced can be put into a dark spray bottle to be used. Using a dark colored bottle will help the solution to remain fresh, which will be felt by the person using it when they apply it to their skin.

3. **Rainfall**

This is another recipe that may be worth trying out. Again, you will need distilled water, some vodka, Sandalwood, Bergamot and Cassis essential oils.

a. 2 cups distilled water
b. 3 tablespoons vodka
c. 5 drops sandalwood
d. 10 drops bergamot
e. 10 drops cassis

These ingredients should be stirred together and then stored overnight in a covered container. Then, the next day, it can be transferred to a dark colored bottle. This perfume must be kept in a cool place so that it does not dry up.

The three perfumes above normally last for about a month before they lose their scent and the next recipe should produce something a bit better.

4. **Inspirational Love**

For next recipe, you will need fragrance oils such as Sandalwood, Cedar Wood, Bergamot, Vodka and a little touch of Vanilla. All these ingredients should be put into a jar and then shaken. It should then be put in a cool place and left for a week. After this time, you can then transfer the mixture into small perfume bottles.

a.   3 drops sandalwood
b.   2 drops vanilla
c.   3 drops Cedar wood
d.   15 drops bergamot
e.   1 cup vodka

If you would like to learn more about recipes for making your own perfume, you could always do a search of the internet. I also recommend visiting your local bookstore, where they will have books on the subject.

It is important to remember that these types of perfume recipes only have a shelf life of a month; therefore you will need to make new batches every few weeks.

CHAPTER 7
CREATING AROMATHERAPY PERFUMES

Using essential oils to make your own perfume is not only great fun, but also extremely satisfying as well. These natural perfumes can help to enhance a person's good mood, drive away a bad one, and help them to relax or even to provide them with some energy. It may even make you feel glamorous, exotic, confident or utterly feminine as well.

The recipes provided below are simple to make and easy to follow, and all you need to do is choose which one you want to try. If you want you could do a search to see which essential oils blend well together. So, by following the simple instructions provided below, you will soon be making your very own aromatherapy perfume.

First, you need a base. It can either be alcohol or carrier oil but the best is a mixture of the two together. The best type of alcohol to use is one which is odorless. Vodka is a good choose and mix this with Jojoba. Jojoba is particularly good, as it has a long shelf life, and once it is put on the skin, it tends to dry out and leave a wonderful scent behind.

Jojoba is one of the more expensive carrier oils, and I would suggest you experiment with one of the cheaper ones like as almond or apricot kernel oil instead. Once you are happy with the product you are producing, you can produce the same product but with jojoba oil instead.

The equipment you will need for making aromatherapy perfume is as follows:-

1.   Measuring Spoons
2.   Small Funnel
3.   Small Colored Bottles
4.   Dropper

Now we will provide you with the instructions for producing your first batch of aromatherapy perfume.

1.   1 teaspoon of carrier oil (Jojoba, Almond or Apricot Kernel) and 1 teaspoon of alcohol (Vodka), and with the small funnel, place these in the bottle.

2.   Next, add the essential oils from your chosen recipe (below you will see a number of different recipes, with the quantities of essential oils you require for them). You may need to get a dropper, as not all essential oil bottles come with one, and add a drop at a time.

3.   After adding each drop of essential oil to the rest of the mixture, the bottle should be shaken (remember to put the lid on first before shaking).

4.   Once you have finished adding the last drops of essential oil and shaken, make sure the lid is on tightly, and

store in a cool dark place for 12 days or more. However, each day you should remember to give the bottles a shake at least 3 times.

5.   After 12 days you can begin to enjoy the aromatherapy perfume that you have made.

The first recipe below is specifically for those women who may suffer from nerves on their wedding day, and will help to feel much more relaxed and calm on their big day.

1.   **Relaxation**

a.   4 drops Jasmine
b.   2 drops Lemon
c.   1 drop Patchouli

The following recipes have been designed to help produce a much more calming effect to the person using them. These perfumes will help to focus you on your inner self, and provide you with a feeling of security, which will promote a feeling of total relaxation.

2.   **Tranquil**

a.   4 drops of Cedar wood
b.   2 drops of Clary Sage
c.   1 drop of Grapefruit
d.   2 drops of Mandarin

3.   **Relax**

a.   2 drops of Grapefruit
b.   2 drops of Patchouli
c.   1 drop of Rose
d.   3 drops of Vetivert
e.   2 drops of Ylang-Ylang

4.   **Sleepy**

a.   2 drops of Bergamot
b.   3 drops of Chamomile
c.   2 drops of Marjoram
d.   4 drops of Lavender

5.   **Silencer**

a.   3 drops of lavender
b.   3 drops of Neroli
c.   2 drops of Spearmint

The next recipes we are looking at will enhance a person's mood and feelings of wellbeing. These perfumes will help to relax and surround you with warmth, as well as a feeling of pure luxury for those special nights out or at home with your loved one.

6.   **Armor**

a.   3 drops of Jasmine
b.   3 drops of Neroli
c.   4 drops of Orange

7.   **Devotional**

a.   1 drop of Clary Sage
b.   3 drop of Patchouli
c.   2 drops of Rose
d.   4 drops of Rosewood

8.   **Tender**

a.   2 drops of Linden Blossom

b.   3 drops of Lime
c.   2 drops of Neroli
d.   3 drops of Sandalwood

9.   **Zingy**

a.   4 drops of Melissa
b.   2 drops of Rose
c.   2 drops of Ylang-Ylang

The long lists of recipes are great collection to have. A couple of the recipes are though colleagues with great testimonials.

10.   **Floral Nights**

a.   2tbsp. jojoba oil
b.   3 drops bergamot oil
c.   2 drops Neroli oil
d.   8 drops jasmine oil
e.   12 drops geranium oil
f.   8 drops ylang-ylang oil
g.   4 drops patchouli oil

11.   **Citrus Drive**

a.   5 tsp. vodka
b.   1/2 tsp. distilled water
c.   15 drops lemon oil
d.   10 drops bergamot oil
e.   10 drops bitter-orange oil
f.   5 drops grapefruit oil
g.   5 drops lemongrass oil
h.   4 drops benzoin oil
i.   2 drops cedar wood oil

12.   In Suspension

a.   2 drops Basil
b.   3 drops Bergamot
c.   1 drop Coriander
d.   4 drops Petitgrain

13.   Fresh Decision

a.   2 drops Benzoin
b.   3 drops Frankincense
c .   1 drop Geranium
d.   3 drops Orange

14.   Self-Impression

a.   2 drops Ginger
b.   3 drops Myrtle
c.   4 drops Rosemary
d.   3 drops Verbena

15.   Happiness

a.   2 drops Bergamot
b.   1 drops Jasmine
c.   1 drops Rose
d.   2 drops Sandalwood

16.   Enjoy Life

a.   2 drops Basil
b.   1 drops Geranium
c.   3 drops Melissa
d.   2 drops Sandalwood

17. Winter Night

a. 2 drops Black Pepper
b. 3 drops Patchouli
c. 4 drops Rosewood
d. 3 drops Ylang-ylang

18. Arabian Breeze

a. 3 drops Coriander
b. 1 drop Frankincense
c. 3 drops Juniper
d. 4 drops Orange

19. Egyptian Night

a. 2 drops Cinnamon
b. 3 drops Lime
c. 4 drops Rose
d. 5 drops Ylang-ylang

20. African Express

a. 3 drops Bergamot
b. 2 drops Palmarosa
c. 3 drops Rose
d. 4 drops Sandalwood

21. Meaningful Thoughts

a. 2 drops Caraway
b. 2 drops Cardamom
c. 2 drops Frankincense
d. 3 drops Rosewood

22. **Divine Fresh**

a. 1 drop Frankincense
b. 4 drops Grapefruit
c. 3 drops Rosemary
d. 2 drops Spearmint

23. **Lift Up**

a. 3 drops Bergamot
b. 1 drop Jasmine
c. 4 drops Lemongrass
d. 1 drops Neroli

24. **Loving Him**

a. 2 drops Coriander
b. 3 drops Lime
c. 4 drops Sandalwood

25. **Loving Her**

a. 3 drops Bergamot
b. 2 drops Jasmine
c. 3 drops Sandalwood

26. **Mother Givens**

a. 3 drops Neroli
b. 3 drops Patchouli
c. 4 drops Rose

27. **Tropic Flower**

a. 10 drops Bergamot

b.   10 drops Lemon
c .   2 drops Rosemary
d.   2 drops Orange
e.   2 drops Neroli

28.   India Xpress

a.   6 drops Sandalwood
b.   5 drops Rose
c.   2 drops Lemon
d.   2 drops Coriander

29.   Old Fashion Romance

a.   12 drops Patchouli
b.   3 drops Geranium
c.   2 drops Ylang-ylang
d.   1 drops Cinnamon

30.   Country Garden Wind

a.   4 drops Rose
b.   2 drops Lemon
c.   2 drops Orange
d.   2 drops Bergamot
e.   1 drops Basil
f.   1 drops Neroli
g.   1 drops Petitgraine

31.   Citrus Spice Breeze

a.   4 drops Bergamot
b.   4 drops Lemon
c.   4 drops Orange
d.   2 drops Rosemary
e.   2 drops Petitgraine
f.   1 drops Rose

32. **Fresh Garden**

a. 10 drops Palmarosa
b. 8 drops Orange
c. 3 drops Petitgraine
d. 2 drops Lime
e. 1 drop Geranium

33. **Living it Up**

a. 9 drops Grapefruit
b. 5 drops Clary Sage
c. 3 drops Geranium

34. **Exotic Spin**

a. 12 drops Rosewood
b. 6 drops Ylang-ylang
c. 2 drops Jasmine

35. **Romantic Night**

a. 2 drops sandalwood
b. 2 drops patchouli
c. 2 drops Ylang-ylang

36. **Serenity Fresh**

a. 2 drops sandalwood
b. 2 drops Ylang-ylang
c. 2 drops valerian

37. **Sprit Scent**

a. 2 drops sandalwood
b. 2 drops bergamot

c.   2 drops juniper

38.   Teen Love

a.   2 drops sandalwood
b.   2 drops vetiver
c.   2 drops rosewood

39.   Mystery Side

a.   8 drops Sandalwood
b.   3 drops Lavender
c.   1 drop Cedar wood

40.   Floral Romance

a.   5 drops Palmarosa
b.   3 drops Rosewood
c.   1 drop Rose Geranium
d.   1 drop Ylang-ylang

41.   Youngness

a.   9 drops Grapefruit
b.   1 drop Rose Geranium
c.   1 drop Ylang-ylang

42.   Lavender Wisp

a.   6 drops Lavender
b.   4 drops Frankincense
c.   1 drop Rosewood

43. Rose Garden Touch

a. 6 drops Rose
b. 3 drops Rosewood
c. 1 drop Jasmine

44. Rose Garden Twist

a. 6 drops Rose
b. 3 drops Rosewood
c. 1 drop Ylang-ylang

45. Spicy Essence

a. 8 drops Sandalwood
b. 2 drops Orange
c. 1 drop Patchouli
d. 1 drop Ylang-ylang

46. Sweet Twist

a. 5 drops Vanilla
b. 4 drops Cocoa Absolute
c. 1 drop Ylang-ylang

47. Morning After

a. 5 drops Bergamot
b. 5 drops Grapefruit
c. 1dropsRoseGeraniu

CHAPTER 8
SIMPLE PERFUMES AND BODY SPRAYS

In this chapter we will look at a number of different recipes, not just for perfumes, but colognes and body sprays as well, which all can easily be made in your own home.

The first recipe we will be looking at is the basic perfume recipe. This is the simplest of all perfume recipes that you can reproduce at home.

Ingredients
1.   2 cups of water
2.   2 cup fresh chopped flower blossoms (you may want to use such flowers as lavender, lilac, orange blossoms or honeysuckle).

Directions
1.   In a bowl, put a cheesecloth (make sure that the edges of the cloth hang over the side of the bowl). Fill this with 1 cup of flower blossoms (you choose) and then pour water over them until they are completely covered.
2.   Cover the bowl and allow it to sit overnight. The following day, take hold of the edges of the cheesecloth hanging over the side of the bowl and lift it up, then gently squeeze the scented water produced into a small pot. You will now need to place this water into a pot and allow it to simmer until there is about 1 teaspoon left of the liquid.

Allow the solution to cool, and place it in a small bottle. Perfume made this way normally has a shelf life of about 1 month.

The following recipes are all as easy to make as the basic recipe, but they will all be a little more fragrant because of the ingredients used. They also include either essential or fragrance oils as part of the recipe.

The first will bring the Orient Side to you.

1. **Orient Side**

a.   4 drops of Sandalwood
b.   4 drops of Musk
c.   3 drops of Frankincense
d.   2 teaspoons of Jojoba oil

Directions
1.   Mix all of the ingredients together in a bottle and shake well.
2.   Place them in a dark colored bottle, and then allow the perfume to settle for at least 12 hours.
3.   Once it has been stood for 12 hours or more, you should now store it in a cool dry area.

The next recipe is also simple to make, but uses not only essential fragrance oils, but also water and alcohol, as previously mentioned in this book.

2. **Sweet Country Garden**

a.   1 cups distilled water
b.   2 tablespoons of Vodka
c.   3 drops of Lavender
d.   5 drops of Chamomile
e.   5 drops of Valerian

f.   1 drop   of Vanilla

Directions
1.   Mix all these ingredients together in a bottle and shake it well.
2.   Transfer the mixture to a dark colored bottle, and again, as with the previous recipe, allow the bottle to stand for 12 hours or more.
3.   Once the bottle has stood for the recommended 12 hours, it can be used, and then stored in a cool dry area.

The next recipe we are looking at is in fact not a perfume, but colognes, and contains lemon as the main ingredient.

1.   **Tropical Breeze**

a.   1 cup of distilled water
b.   1 cup of Vodka
c.   3 drops of Lemongrass
d.   10 drops of Lavender
e.   10 drops of Lime

Directions
1.   Combine the essential oils with the vodka in a bottle and shake well.
2.   Now set this aside for 3 weeks.
3.   After 3 weeks, you will need to add the distilled water and then let it stand for a further week.
4.   It is important that you shake the bottle once a day while it is standing over the 4 week period.
5.   After 4 weeks, you can transfer the mixture to dark bottles for storage, or keep the mixture in the bottle it is in. Store the mixture in a dark cool place.

2. **Confident Style**

a. 1 cup Vodka
b. 3 drops of Everlasting
c. 3 drops of Peony
d. 2 drops of Sandalwood

Directions
1. Combine the essential oils with the vodka in a bottle and shake well.
2. Now set this aside for 1 week

3. **Serenity**

a. 3 drops Bergamot
b. 2 drops Frankincense
c. 3 drops Cedar wood
d. 1 cup of Vodka

Direction

1. Combine the essential oils with the vodka in a bottle and shake well.
2. Now set this aside for 1 week

The final recipe provided below is one which will produce a body splashes, rather than a perfumes.

1. **Tropical Flower**

a.   2 cups of distilled water
b.   3 tablespoons of vodka
c.   1 tablespoon each of finely chopped lemon and orange peel
d.   5 drops of Lemon Verbena
e.   10 drops of Mandarin
f.   10 drops of Orange

Directions
1.   Mix the fruit peels with the vodka in a jar, cover and let it stand for 1 week.
2.   After the week, strain the liquid and add the essential oils and distilled water to it.
3.   Now the mixture stands for a further 2 weeks. Make sure to shake the jar well once a day during this time.
4.   Place the final solution after the 2 weeks in a dark bottle(s), or keep it in a cool dark area.

2.   **Passion Mist**

a.   3 drops passionflower essential/fragrance oil
b.   2 drops Ylang-ylang essential/fragrance oil
c.   3 drops Neroli essential/fragrance oil
d.   3 tablespoons of vodka
e.   1 cup distilled water

Directions
1.   Pour the alcohol into a dark bottle or jar. Add the oils and shake well.
2.   Leave for 1 week. Store in a cool dry area.

3. **Lite Summer Mist**

a.   1 tablespoon witch hazel
b.   1 teaspoon lemon essential/fragrance oil
c.   1 teaspoon cucumber essential/fragrance oil
d.   1 cup water

Directions:
1.   For a refreshing cool feeling, make an after shower spray by combining all the ingredients. Place in a pump spray bottle.

As you can see making your own perfumes, colognes or body sprays is simple. Once you've made your first lot and tried it yourself, you will soon want to be making more.

CHAPTER 9
SELLING YOUR PERFUME

You have now begun to produce your homemade perfume, and have decided not just to give it as gifts to your friends or family, but instead would like to sell it to a wider audience.

One of the first things you will need to look at when making the decision on selling your own perfume is what it will be called. You will then need to start looking for bottles into which you can put your finished perfume. Then you will need to design a label for inclusion on the bottle, you can use any drawing program to make the labels. Think of what kind of packaging that you will present the perfume in.

When looking at what sort of bottles you are considering to place your finished product in, you might want to think about vintage perfume, bottles but make sure they have been thoroughly sterilized? They will certainly provide you with an individual look that cannot be found when buying perfumes that have been mass produced. Just take a wander around your local antique shops, bric-a-brac shop, or online. You will soon find a wealth of different perfume bottles that you could use.

The best place to start when you are considering selling your own perfume is to do a search on the internet. There are many sites and companies which will provide you with all the necessary information you need in order to start up. EBay and Amazon are the top sites to sell on. You should be warned, when you decide to sell your own perfume, you will need to make some outlays in order to get the business started.

You will need to factor in such costs as the purchase of all the ingredients for making the perfume, and the bottles that you will be putting the finished product into. Other costs that you will have to pay out for are the production of the labels that will be affixed to your finished product's bottles, and the cost of the packaging that you will use.

When first selling your product, it is advisable that you keep a record of all of your outgoing expenses so that you can price your perfume accordingly. The usual pricing equation is to triple the price it has cost you to manufacture your product.

One of the best ways of selling your own perfume is through word of mouth of friends and family. You could actually set up your own website and sell it from there. If you are not sure how to go about setting up a website, then by searching the internet you will soon find there are lots of people out there who are willing to help. There are even people who have set up sites which will not only help you to build your site, but also help with the marketing and promotion of the product you have to offer. Begin by doing a search on the internet and looking for "starting a small web business". You will soon find a whole list of sites that are willing to assist you.

CHAPTER 10
DESIGNER NOTES

If you are like me and are interested in designer perfumes or colognes. You might want to try making your own. You might even want to improve on the designer perfume by add a little touch of another scent. Plus you could take the scent and make it into a body spray. It occurred to me that you might want the list perfumes and colognes; in return I include over 50 pages of designer perfume notes and cologne notes.

Adoration
Floral

Top Notes: Freesia
Heart Notes: Apricot blossoms

Alexandra (Alexandra de Mark off)
Semi-Oriental

Top Notes: Italian Iris, South African marigold
Heart Notes: French Jasmine, Moroccan rose, French jonquil
Base Notes: Indian sandalwood, Singapore patchouli, Reunion island vetiver

Aliage (Estee Lauder)
Chypre-Green

Top Notes: Greens, peach, citrus
Heart Notes: Jasmine, rosewood, pine, thyme
Base Notes: Oakmoss, musk, vetiver, myrrh

Alchimie (Rochas)
Floral-Oriental

Top Notes: Blackcurrant, bergamot, grapefruit
Heart Notes: Acacia, jasmin, passiflora
Base Notes: Sandalwood, vanilla, tonka bean

Amarige (Givenchy)
Floral-Fruity

Top Notes: Mandarin, neroli, violet leaves, rosewood
Heart Notes: Gardenia, red fruits, ylang-ylang, acacia farnesiana, mimosa
Base Notes: Musk, vanilla, tonka bean, woods, ambergris

Amazone (Hermes)
Floral-Fruity, this is a dry scent (not too sweet)

Top Notes: Mandarin, neroli, violet leaves, rosewood
Heart Notes: Daffodil, hyacinth, narcissus, black currant bud, iris, jasmine, raspberry, lily of the valley.
Base Notes: Sandalwood, vetiver, cedarwood, neroli, ylang-ylang, oakmoss

Amour Amour (Jean Patou)
Floral-Fresh

Top Notes: Bergamot, strawberry, lemon, neroli

Heart Notes: Jasmine, narcissus, rose, ylang-ylang, carnation, oregano, lily

Base Notes: Vetiver, honey, musk, civet, heliotrope

Anais Anais (Cacharel)
Floral-Fresh

Top Notes: White Madonna lily, black currant bud, hyacinth, lily of the valley, citrus

Heart Notes: Moroccan jasmine, Grasse rose, Florentine Iris, Madagascar ylang-ylang, orange blossom, Bourbon vetiver.

Base Notes: Russian leather, musk

Angel (Thierry Mugler)
Oriental, chocolate-vanilla

Top Notes: Fruits, dewberry, helonial, honey
Heart Notes: Chocolate, caramel, coumarin
Base Notes: Vanilla, patchouli

Animale (Suzanne de Lyon)
Chypre-Floral

Top Notes: Neroli, bergamot, hyacinth, coriander, greens
Heart Notes: Jasmine, rose, pimento berry, ylang-ylang
Base Notes: Patchouli, vetiver, musk, labdanum, oakmoss

Anne Klein
Floral

Top Notes: Greens, galbanum, hyacinth, neroli, cassie, bergamot, aldehydes

Heart Notes: Bulgarian rose, mandarin, lily of the valley, jasmine, orchid, rose

Base Notes: Sandalwood, vetiver, vanilla, amber, benzoin, musk, civet

Anne Klein II
Oriental-Ambery, vanilla

Top Notes: Peach, rosewood, greens, lemon
Heart Notes: Lily, jasmine, rose, orange blossom, ylang-ylang, orris, carnation
Base Notes: Vanilla, amber, sandalwood, musk, patchouli, civet, benzoin

Antilope (Weil)
Floral-Aldehyde

Top Notes: Grasse neroli, bergamot, chamomile, sage, aldehydes
Heart Notes: Lily of the valley, jasmine
Base Notes: Patchouli, iris, ambergris, vetiver

Antonia's Flowers
Floral

Notes: Freesia, jasmine, lily of the valley, magnolia, fruits

Apres L'Ondee (Guerlain)
Floral-Ambery

Top Notes: Violet, bergamot, cassie, neroli
Heart Notes: Carnation, ylang-ylang, iris, rose, jasmine, mimosa, vetiver, sandalwood
Base Notes: Vanilla, musk, amber, heliotrope

Aromatics Elixir
Chypre-Floral

Top Notes: Chamomile, orange blossom, bergamot, coriander, rosewood, aldehydes, greens, palmarosa
Heart Notes: Jasmine, rose, ylang-ylang, tuberose, orris, carnation
Base Notes: Sandalwood, oakmoss, vetiver, patchouli, musk, cistus, civet

Arpege (Lanvin)
Floral-Aldehyde

Top Notes: Bergamot, neroli, aldehydes, peach
Heart Notes: Rose, jasmine, ylang-ylang, lily of the valley
Base Notes: Sandalwood, vetiver, patchouli, vanilla, musk

Asja (Fendi)
Floral-Oriental

Top Notes: Fruits, citrus
Heart Notes: Bulgarian rose, Egyptian jasmine, ylang-ylang, cinnamon, nutmeg, mimosa
Base Notes: Sandalwood, musk, vanilla, amber

Azzaro
Chypre-Fruity

Top Notes: Fruits, gardenias, aldehydes
Heart Notes: Jasmine, rose, ylang-ylang, orris
Base Notes: Moss, styrax, amber, vetiver, patchouli

Azzaro 9
Floral

Top Notes: Pineapple, aldehydes, mandarin, bergamot
Heart Notes: Jasmine, foxglove, tulip, wisteria, clematis, lily, mimosa, rose, orange blossom
Base Notes: Sandalwood, cedarwood, musk, moss, vanilla

Bal A Versailles
Oriental-Ambery Spicy

Top Notes: Grasse jasmine, Bulgarian rose, Anatolian rose, May rose, Farnesian cassie
Heart Notes: Sandalwood, patchouli, vetiver
Base Notes: Musk, ambergris, gums, resins, civet

Balahe (Leonard)
Floral-Ambery

Top Notes: Bergamot, mandarin, clary sage, coriander, pineapple, plum
Heart Notes: Rose, jasmine, ylang-ylang, tuberose, orange blossom, orchid
Base Notes: Vanilla, vetiver, sandalwood, musk, civet

Bandit (Robert Piguet)
Chypre-Floral

Top Notes: Artemisia, bergamot, gardenia, aldehydes
Heart Notes: Jasmine, orris, rose, carnation
Base Notes: Moss, castoreum, patchouli, amber, vetiver, civet, myrrh

Basic Black (Bill Blass)
Floral-Fruity

Top Notes: Bergamot, mandarin, ylang-ylang, cardamon
Heart Notes: Rose, violet, coriander
Base Notes: Patchouli, oakmoss, sandalwood
Beautiful (Estee Lauder)
Floral
Top Notes: Bergamot, galbanum, lemon, cassie, fruits
Heart Notes: Rose, ylang-ylang, lilac, violet, lily of the valley, carnation, sage, geranium, rose violet, narcissus,

orange blossom, mimosa, marigold, freesia, chamomile, tuberose, jasmine, neroli, jonquil, magnolia
Base Notes: Sandalwood, vetiver, musk, vanilla, cedarwood

Bellodgia (Caron)
Floral

Top Notes: Rose, jasmine, lily of the valley
Base Notes: Spicy carnation

Bijan
Floral-Oriental

Top Notes: Ylang-ylang, narcissus, orange blossom
Heart Notes: Persian jasmine, Bulgarian rose, lily of the valley
Base Notes: Moroccan oakmoss, sandalwood, patchouli

Bill Blass
Floral

Top Notes: Galbanum, hyacinth, pineapple, greens, bergamot, geranium
Heart Notes: Iris, tuberose, carnation, ylang-ylang, orris
Base Notes: Amber, sandalwood, benzoin, cedarwood, oakmoss

Blue Grass
Elizabeth Arden

Top Notes: Aldehydes, lavender, orange, neroli, bergamot
Heart Notes: Jasmine, tuberose, narcissus, rose, carnation
Base Notes: Sandalwood, musk, tonka bean, benzoin

Bois de Iles (Chanel)

Floral-Aldehyde

Top Notes: Bergamot, petitgrain, coriander, aldehydes
Heart Notes: Jasmine, rose, ylang-ylang, iris
Base Notes: Vetiver, amber, sandalwood, tonka bean

Boucheron
Floral Semi-Oriental

Top Notes: Sicilian tangerine, Calabrian bitter orange,
apricot, Persian galbanum, African tegetes, Spanish basilica
Heart Notes: Morrocan orange blossom, Grasse
tuberose, Madagascar ylang-ylang, Moroccan jasmine,
Auvergne narcissus, British broom
Base Notes: Mysore sandalwood, amber, Indian Ocean
vanilla, South American tonka bean

Bvlgari
Floral

Top Notes: Italian bergamot, Spanish orange blossom,
Ceylonese cardamom, Jamaican pepper, Russian coriander
Heart Notes: Bulgarian rose, Egyptian jasmine
Base Notes: Green tea, woods

Byblos
Floral-Fruity

Top Notes: Mandarin, grapefruit, cassie, marigold,
bergamot, peach
Heart Notes: Honeysuckle, gardenia, mimosa, ylang-
ylang, lily of the valley, orchid, rose, heliotrope, violet, orris
Base Notes: Musk, vetiver, pepper, raspberry

Byzance (Rochas)
Floral Semi-Oriental

Top Notes: Citrus, cardamon, spices, greens, mandarin, aldehydes, basil

Heart Notes: Jasmine, tuberose, Turkish rose, lily of the valley, ylang-ylang

Base Notes: Sandalwood, vanilla, musk, heliotrope, amber

C'est la Vie (Christian Lacroix)
Floral-Ambery

Top Notes: Bergamot, orange blossom, pineapple, peach, aldehydes

Heart Notes: Ylang-Ylang, carnation, jasmine, rose, tuberose, heliotrope, orris

Base Notes: Amber, vanilla, cedarwood, sandalwood, musk

Cabochard (Gres)
Chypre-Floral

Top Notes: Citrus, aldehydes, fruits, spices

Heart Notes: Jasmine, rose, ylang-ylang, orris, geranium

Base Notes: Leather, tobacco, amber, patchouli, musk, moss, vetiver, castoreum

Cabotine (Gres)
Floral-Green

Top Notes: Orange blossom, tangerine, ylang-ylang, peach, plum, greens, cassie, coriander

Heart Notes: Ginger lily, iris, hyacinth, tuberose, rose, carnation, jasmine, heliotrope

Base Notes: Sandalwood, black currant bud, musk, vanilla, amber, cedarwood, civet, vetiver, tonka bean

Caesars Woman
Floral-Ambery

Top Notes: Orange blossom, geranium
Heart Notes: Egyptian jasmine, rose, iris
Base Notes: Tibetan musk, sandalwood, patchouli

Calandre (Paco Rabanne)
Floral-Aldehyde

Top Notes: Greens, aldehydes, bergamot
Heart Notes: Rose, jasmine, lily of the valley, geranium, orris
Base Notes: Sandalwood, vetiver, oakmoss, amber, musk

Caleche (Hermes)
Floral-Aldehyde

Top Notes: Bergamot, lemon, aldehydes, neroli
Heart Notes: Gardenia, ylang-ylang, jasmine, rose, iris
Base Notes: Sandalwood, oakmoss, cedarwood, vetiver, amber, musk

Calyx (Prescriptives)
Floral-Fruity

Top Notes: Passion fruit, mango, pamplemousse, mandarin, guava, papaya
Heart Notes: Lily, neroli, jasmine, freesia, rose, marigold, lily of the valley, melon
Base Notes: Cedarwood, moss, musk, raspberry

Capricci (Nina Ricci)
Floral

Top Notes: Bergamot, greens
Heart Notes: Bulgarian rose, May rose, hyacinth, jasmine, gardenia, ylang-ylang, geranium, lily of the valley, narcissus, tuberose, orris
Base Notes: Vetiver, sandalwood, musk, moss, benzoin

Carolina Herrera
Floral

Top Notes: Orange blossom, apricot, rosewood, bergamot, greens

Heart Notes: French and Spanish jasmine, Indian tuberose, hyacinth, honeysuckle, narcissus, ylang-ylang, lily of the valley

Base Notes: Amber, moss, sandalwood, cedarwood, vetiver, musk, civet

Casmir (Chopard)
Oriental-Fruity (Vanilla theme)

Top Notes: Peach, mango, coconut, bergamot, hesperides

Heart Notes: Jasmine, lily of the valley, geranium

Base Notes: Vanilla, amber, sandalwood, patchouli, castoreum, musk

Cassini (Oleg Cassini)
Chypre-Fruity floral

Top Notes: Mandarin, freesia, osmanthus

Heart Notes: Jasmine, Bulgarian rose, tuberose, chrysanthemum, carnation

Base Notes: Mousse de chene, amber, oakmoss

Catalyst (Halston)
Floral

Top Notes: Jonquil, tuberose, otto of rose, jasmine absolute, galbanum

Heart Notes: Black currant bud, lily of the valley, violet, chamomile, herbs

Base Notes: Vetiver, sandalwood, patchouli, oakmoss, musk

Chamade (Guerlain)
Floral Semi-Oriental

Top Notes: Greens, galbanum, bergamot, hyacinth, aldehydes

Heart Notes: Rose, jasmine, lilac, clove

Base Notes: Vanilla, amber, benzoin, sandalwood, vetiver

Champagne (YSL) (This fragrance is now called Yvresse)
Floral-Fruity

Top Notes: Nectarine, mint, anise
Heart Notes: Blue rose, otto rose, lychee
Base Notes: Oakmoss, vetiver, patchouli

Chanel No.5
Floral-Aldehyde

Top Notes: Aldehydes, Grasse jasmine
Heart Notes: Rose, ylang-ylang, iris
Base Notes: Amber, patchouli

Chanel No.19
Floral-Green

Top Notes: Greens, galbanum, bergamot
Heart Notes: Jasmine, May rose, iris, ylang-ylang
Base Notes: Sandalwood, oakmoss, vetiver

Chanel No.22
Floral

Notes: White roses, jasmine, tuberose, lily of the valley, lilac, orange blossom

Chant D'Aromes (Guerlain)
Chypre-Floral

Top Notes: Mirabelle, gardenia, aldehydes, fruits
Heart Notes: Rose, jasmine, honeysuckle, ylang-ylang
Base Notes: Benzoin, musk, vetiver, heliotrope, moss, olibanum

Chantilly (Houbigant)
Oriental-Ambery

Top Notes: Fruits, lemon, bergamot, neroli
Heart Notes: Jasmine, rose, orange blossom, spices, ylang-ylang, carnation
Base Notes: Indian sandalwood, moss, vanilla, musk, leather, tonka bean, benzoin

Charles of the Ritz (now called Ritz)
Floral-Oriental

Top Notes: Orange blossom, bergamot, lemon, pineapple
Heart Notes: Jasmine, tuberose, gardenia, neroli, geranium, rose, orris, carnation, lilac, ylang-ylang
Base Notes: Sandalwood, coriander, patchouli, vanilla, vetiver, musk, cedarwood, amber, cinnamon
Chloe (Karl Lagerfeld)

Floral

Top Notes: Honeysuckle, orange blossom, hyacinth, ylang-ylang, lilac

Heart Notes: Tuberose, jasmine, narcissus, carnation, orris, rose

Base Notes: Amber, sandalwood, oakmoss

Chloe Narcisse (Karl Lagerfeld)

Floral-Oriental

Top Notes: Orange blossom, apricot, plumeria, marigold

Heart Notes: Jasmine, rose otto, narcissus, spices

Base Notes: Sandalwood, vanilla absolute, musk, tolu balsam

Ciara (Revlon)

Oriental-Ambery

Top Notes: Vanilla, sandalwood, patchouli, cedarwood

Heart Notes: Herbaceous spices

Base Notes: Frankincense, balsam, myrrh, raspberry

Cinnabar (Estee Lauder)

Oriental-Spicy

Top Notes: Tangerine, orange blossom, clove, peach, bergamot, spices

Heart Notes: Jasmine, rose, carnation, ylang-ylang

Base Notes: Amber, patchouli, incense, vanilla, vetiver, benzoin, tolu

Coeur-Joie (Nina Ricci)

Floral

Top Notes: Neroli, bergamot

Heart Notes: Florentine Iris, Oriental rose, jasmine, violet

Base Notes: Woods

Colors (Benetton)

Semi-Oriental

Top Notes: Moroccan orange blossom, French hyacinth, Egyptian marigold, Isreali basil

Heart Notes: Comoros Island tuberose, French jasmine, Hawaiian pineapple, Caribbean passion fruit, Georgia peach, Bulgarian rose.

Base Notes: Madagascar vanilla, Yugoslavian oakmoss, Chinese patchouli, Virginian cedarwood, Ethiopian civet, opopanax

Coriandre (Jean Couturier)
Chypre-Floral

Top Notes: Coriander, aldehydes, orange blossom, angelica
Heart Notes: Rose, geranium, l;ily, jasmine, orris
Base Notes: Sandalwood, vetiver, musk, oakmoss, patchouli

Coriolan (Guerlain)
Citrus-Woods

Top Notes: Citrus, bergamot, lemon leaf, neroli, sage
Heart Notes: Absinthe, ylang-ylang, sandalwood, basil, pepper, coriander, ginger, juniper berries
Base Noes: Vetiver, patchouli, spicebush

Courreges in Blue
Floral

Top Notes: French marigold, basil, bergamot, mandarin, geranium, coriander, aldehydes
Heart Notes: Rose, jasmine, black currant bud, peach, peony, violet, orange blossom, tuberose
Base Notes: Sandalwood, clove, patchouli, vetiver, cedarwood, civet, musk, amber, moss

Creation (Ted Lapidus)
Chypre-Fresh

Top Notes: Black currant bud, mango, passion fruit, peach, bergamot, lemon, mandarin, galbanum

Heart Notes: Gardenia, jasmine, tuberose, narcissus, rose, ylang-ylang, carnation, lily of the valley

Base Notes: Amber, oakmoss, musk, sandalwood, patchouli, vanilla, civet

Cristalle (Chanel)
Chypre-Fresh

Top Notes: Greens, mandarin, lemon, bergamot, galbanum, basil, lavender

Heart Notes: Rose, hyacinth, honeysuckle, jasmine, peach, lily of the valley, ylang-ylang, iris, mosses

Base Notes: Woods, santal, musk, fruits, sandalwood, oakmoss

Cuir de Russie (Chanel)
Chypre-Floral

Top Notes: Orange blossom, bergamot, mandarin, clary sage

Heart Notes: Iris, jasmine, rose, ylang-ylang, cedarwood, vetiver

Base Notes: Balsamics, leather, amber, vanilla

Delicious (Gale Hayman)
Floral

Top Notes: Narcisse, mimosa, mandarin, boronia, neroli, black currant bud

Heart Notes: Rose, jasmine, tuberose, lily of the valley, ylang-ylang, angelica

Base Notes: Sandalwood, patchouli, musk, orris

Demi-Jour (Houbigant)
Floral

Top Notes: Bergamot, aldehydes, greens, violet
Heart Notes: Rose, orris, lily of the valley, jasmine, ylang-ylang, heliotrope
Base Notes: Musk, moss, sandalwood, cedarwood

Design (Paul Sebastian)
Floral-Fruity

Top Notes: Peach, orange blossom, jasmine, tuberose
Heart Notes: Gardenia, lilac, honeysuckle, carnation
Base Notes: Black currant bud, musk, sandalwood, civet

Desirade (Aubusson)
Floral Semi-Oriental

Top Notes: Italian bergamot, Russian coriander, Madagascar ylang-ylang, pineapple, aldehydes
Heart Notes: Chinese osmanthus, jasmine, rose, cassia, tuberose, orange blossom, violet
Base Notes: Sandalwood, patchouli, vetiver, Somalian opopanax, plum, raspberry, vanilla, musk

Destiny (Marilyn Miglin)
Floral-Fresh

Notes: Calla lilies, white rose, fo-ti-tieng, osmanthus, karo karunde, white orchid, narcissus

Di Borghese
Floral-Oriental

Top Notes: Greens, moss
Heart Notes: Jasmine, hyacinth, lily of the valley, narcissus
Base Notes: Amber, sandalwood, spices

Diamonds and Emeralds (Elizabeth Taylor)

Floral

Top Notes: Gardenia, white rose, apricot, tangerine, peach, sage, hyacinth, orange blossom, greens
Heart Notes: Jasmine, lily of the valley, carnation, rose, tuberose, magnolia, wild lily
Base Notes: Vanilla, amber, musk, patchouli, vetiver, tonka bean

Diamonds and Rubies (Elizabeth Taylor)
Floral-Oriental

Top Notes: Peach, red rose, Amazon lily, French lilac, peach, bitter almond
Heart Notes: Jasmine, cattleya orchid, heliotrope, spices, rose, ylang-ylang, wild lily of the valley
Base Notes: Amber, cedarwood, vanilla, benzoin, musk, sandalwood

Diamonds and Sapphires (Elizabeth Taylor)
Floral-Fruity

Top Notes: Freesia, lily of the valley, melon, peach, galbanum
Heart Notes: Rose, jasmine, rhubrum lily, ylang-ylang, spices, tagetes
Base Notes: Sandalwood, vetiver, amber, musk

Dilys (Laura Ashley)
Floral

Top Notes: Orange Blossom, neroli, narcissus
Heart Notes: Moroccan rose, French jasmine, tuberose, ylang-ylang, lily of the valley
Base Notes: Sandalwood, musk, oakmoss
Diorella (Christian Dior)
Chypre-Fresh

Top Notes: Sicilian lemon, greens, basil, Italian bergamot, melon

Heart Notes: Moroccan jasmine, rose, carnation, cyclamen

Base Notes: Oakmoss, vetiver, musk, patchouli

Dioressence (Christian Dior)

Oriental-Spicy

Top Notes: Aldehydes, greens, fruits

Heart Notes: Jasmine, geranium, cinnamon, carnation, tuberose, ylang-ylang, orris

Base Notes: Patchouli, oakmoss, vetiver, benzoin, vanilla, musk, styrax

Diorissimo (Christian Dior)

Floral-Fresh

Top Notes: Greens, bergamot, calyx

Heart Notes: Lily of the valley, jasmine, boronia, rosewood, ylang-ylang, lilac

Base Notes: Sandalwood, civet

Diva (Ungaro)

Chypre-Floral

Top Notes: Mandarin, ylang-ylang, Indian tuberose, cardamon, bergamot, coriander, aldehydes

Heart Notes: Honeyed Moroccan rose, Turkish rose, Egyptian jasmine, Florentine iris, narcissus, carnation, orris

Base Notes: Patchouli, ambergris, oakmoss, sandalwood, vetiver, musk, civet, honey

DNA (Bijan)

Floral-Ambery

Top Notes: Rosewood, minty geranium, ylang-ylang, bergamot

Heart Notes: Jasmine, lily of the valley, tuberose, clove, osmanthus

Base Notes: Myrrh, oakmoss, sandalwood, vetiver, vanilla, benzoin, amber

Dolce & Gabbana

Floral-Oriental

Top Notes: Tangerine, basil, ivy, freesia, petitgrain
Heart Notes: Bulgarian rose, marigold, lily of the valley, orange blossom, red carnation, jasmine, coriander
Base Notes: Sandalwood, tonka bean, vanilla, musk

Donna Karan New York
Floral

Top Notes: Casablanca lily, apricot
Heart Notes: Rose, cassia, ylang-ylang, jasmine, heliotrope
Base Notes: Suede, amber, sandalwood, patchouli

Dune (Christian Dior)
Floral

Notes: Lily, wallflower, peony, amber, broom, lichen

Eau D'Hadrien (Annick Goutal)
Chypre-Fresh

Notes: Sicilian lemon, grapefruit, citron, cypress

Eau D'Hermes (Hermes)
Floral-Fruity

Top Notes: Cardamom, herbal lavender, petitgrain lemon, cinnamon, cumin
Heart Notes: Jasmine, Bourbon geranium, vanilla, tonka bean, labdanum
Base Notes: Sandalwood, cedarwood, flamed birch

Eau de Camille (Anick Goutal)
Floral-Green
Notes: Honeysuckle, ivy, grass, seringa

Eau de Charlotte (Annick Goutal)

Floral-Fruity

Notes: Mimosa, black currant bud, cocoa, lily of the valley

Eau de Cologne du Coq (Guerlain)
Citrus

Top Notes: Hesperides, lemon, bergamot, neroli
Heart Notes: Lavender, jasmine, patchouli
Base Notes: Moss, sandalwood

Eau de Cologne Hermes
Citrus
Top Notes: Mint, mango, papaya, buchu bark, lemon, mandarin, bergamot, basil, coriander
Heart Notes: Neroli, orange leaves, lily of the valley, honeysuckle, lavender, rosemary
Base Notes: Petitgrain citron, oakmoss, patchouli, musk, cedarwood, sandalwood

Eau de Cologne Imperiale (Guerlain)
Citrus

Top Notes: Hesperides, orange blossom, bergamot, neroli, lemon
Heart Notes: Lavender
Base Notes: Rosemary, tonka bean, cedarwood

Eau de Givenchy
Floral-Fruity

Top Notes: Bergamot, spearmint, tagetes, greens, fruits
Heart Notes: Jasmine, lily of the valley, rose, cyclamen, orris
Base Notes: Musk, cedarwood, sandalwood, moss

Eau de Gucci
Floral-Fresh

Top Notes: Mandarin, ylang-ylang, greens, bergamot, hyacinth, lemon
Heart Notes: Jasmine, lilac, lily of the valley, honeysuckle, orris, tuberose, rose
Base Notes: Cedarwood, amber, musk, vetiver, moss, sandalwood

Eau de Guerlain
Citrus

Top Notes: Lemon, bergamot, basil, petitgrain, fruits, caraway
Heart Notes: Thyme, mint, lavender, jasmine, carnation, patchouli, rose, sandalwood
Base Notes: Moss, amber, musk

Eau de Patou (Jean Patou)
Citrus

Top Notes: Sicilian citron, Guinea oranges, Grasse petitgrain
Heart Notes: Tunisian orange blossom, pepper, nasturtium, honeysuckle, ylang-ylang
Base Notes: Musk, moss, amber, civet, labdanum

Eau de Rochas
Chypre-Fresh

Top Notes: Sicilian lime, Calabrian mandarin, bergamot, tangerine, grapefruit
Heart Notes: Wild rose, mountain narcissus
Base Notes: Mysore sandalwood, Croatian oakmoss, amber

Eau de Ciel (Annick Goutal)
Floral

Notes: Brazilian rosewood, iris, violet

Eau Fraiche (Leonard)
Citrus

Top Notes: Italian bergamot, mandarin, Sicilian lemon
Heart Notes: Florals, clove, coriander
Base Notes: Haitian vetiver, Singapore patchouli

Ellen Tracy
Floral

Top Notes: Peach, galbanum, osmanthus, hyacinth
Heart Notes: Jasmine, tuberose, rose, ylang-ylang
Base Notes: Sandalwood, moss, amber

Elysium (Clarins)
Floral-Fruity

Top Notes: Jasmine, honeydew, ylang-ylang, dewberry, linden blossom
Heart Notes: Lily of the valley, freesia, rose, osmanthus
Base Notes: Sandalwood, papaya, musk, cedarwood

Empreinte (Courreges)
Chypre-Floral

Top Notes: Peach, bergamot, coriander, artemisia, aldehydes
Heart Notes: Bulgarian rose, Grasse jasmine, melon, orris
Base Notes: Amber, patchouli, oakmoss, cedarwood, sandalwood, castoreum

Enigma (Alexandra de Markoff)

Chypre

Top Notes: Aldehydes, greens, bergamot, coriander, pimento, herbs
Heart Notes: Jasmine, rose, carnation
Base Notes: Amber, woods, spices, patchouli, oakmoss

Escada
Floral-Oriental

Top Notes: Bergamot, hyacinth, peach, coconut
Heart Notes: Orange blossom, jasmine, iris, carnation, frangipani flower
Base Notes: Vanilla, musk, sandalwood

Escape (Calvin Klein)
Floral-Fruity

Top Notes: Mandarin, apple, black currant bud, chamomile, apricot, melon, peach, plum
Heart Notes: Jasmine, rose, coriander, clove, carnation
Base Notes: Sandalwood, musk, cedarwood, oakmoss, amber

Estee (Estee Lauder)
Floral

Top Notes: Peach, raspberry, citrus oils
Heart Notes: Rose, lily of the valley, jasmine, carnation, ylang-ylang, honey, orris
Base Notes: Cedarwood, musk, moss, sandalwood, styrax

Eternity (Calvin Klein)
Floral-Fresh

Top Notes: Mandarin, freesia, sage

Heart Notes: Narcissus, lily of the valley, marigold, white lily, jasmine, rose

Base Notes: Sandalwood, patchouli, amber, musk

Farouche (Nina Ricci)
Floral-Aldehyde

Top Notes: Bergamot, mandarin, galbanum, aldehydes, peach

Heart Notes: Rose, jasmine, honeysuckle, clary sage, cardamon, genista flowers, iris, carnation, geranium, lily of the valley, lily

Base Notes: Oakmoss, sandalwood, amber, vetiver, musk

Feminite du Bois (Shiseido)
Chypre

Top Notes: Cedarwood, orange blossom, peach, honey, plum, beeswax

Heart Notes: Cedarwood, clove, cardamom, cinnamon

Base Notes: Cedarwood, musk

Femme (Rochas)
Chypre-Fruity

Top Notes: Peach, plum, bergamot, lemon, rosewood

Heart Notes: Ylang-ylang, jasmine, May rose, clove, orris

Base Notes: Musk, amber, oakmoss, vanilla, patchouli, benzoin, leather

Fendi
Chypre-Floral

Top Notes: Bergamot, aldehydes, rosewood, fruits

Heart Notes: Jasmine, rose, ylang-ylang, geranium, carnation

Base Notes: Patchouli, musk, leather, sandalwood, cedarwood, spices, amber, vanilla

Ferre 20 (Gianfranco Ferre)

Top Notes: Bergamot, mandarin
Heart Notes: Rose, jasmine, blackberry
Base Notes: Vanilla, musk

Ferre by Ferre (Gianfranco Ferre)
Floral-Fruity
Top Notes: Orange blossom, bergamot, ylang-ylang, butterbush
Heart Notes: Rose, mimosa, peach, passion fruit, violet, cassia, moss, lily of the valley
Base Notes: Vanilla, sandalwood, spices, amber, iris, vetiver, musk

Fidji (Guy Laroche)
Floral

Top Notes: Galbanum, hyacinth, lemon, bergamot
Heart Notes: Carnation, orris, ylang-ylang, jasmine, rose
Base Notes: Vetiver, musk, moss, sandalwood

First (Van Cleef & Arpels)
Floral-Aldehyde

Top Notes: Aldehydes, mandarin, black currant bud, peach, raspberry, hyacinth
Heart Notes: Turkish rose, narcissus, jasmine, lily of the valley, carnation, orchid, tuberose, orris
Base Notes: Amber, tonka bean, oakmoss, sandalwood, vetiver, musk, honey, civet

Fleur D'Eau (Rochas)
Fruity-Floral

Top Notes: Apricot, melon, black currant bud
Heart Notes: Rose, mimosa, heliotrope, lotus, water hyacinth, seringa
Base Notes: Sandalwood, vetiver, amber

Fleur de Fleur (Nina Ricci)
Floral-Aldehyde

Top Notes: Bergamot, greens, lemon, aldehydes
Heart Notes: May rose, Grasse jasmine, iris, hyacinth, ylang-ylang, lily of the valley, lilac, cyclamen, magnolia
Base Notes: Sandalwood, civet, musk

Fleurs de Rocaille (Caron)
Floral

Top Notes: Gardenia, Violet
Heart Notes: Lily of the valley, rose, jasmine, ylang-ylang, lilac, mimosa, iris
Base Notes: Sandalwood, Cedarwood, Amber

Flirt (Prescriptives)

Top Notes: Indonesian dossina, iced pomegranate, leaf greens
Heart Notes: Ginger flower, magnolia, tilleil de Nantes
Base Notes: Madagascar iris, tamboti, woods

Folavril (Annick Goutal)
Floral-Fruity

Notes: Jasmine, mango

4711 Eau de Cologne
Chypre-Fresh

Top Notes: Bergamot, orange oil, lemon, basil, peach
Heart Notes: Bulgarian rose, jasmine, melon, lily, cyclamen
Base Notes: Haitian vetiver, Indian sandalwood, oakmoss, patchouli, cedarwood, musk

Fracas (Robert Piguet)
Floral

Top Notes: Bergamot, peach, orange blossom, greens
Heart Notes: Tuberose, rose, jasmine, carnation, orris
Base Notes: Sandalwood, cedarwood, moss, musk

Gardenia Passion (Annick Goutal)
Floral

Notes: Gardenia

Gem (Van Cleef & Arpels)
Chypre-Fruity

Top Notes: Peach, plum, myrtle, cypress, cardamon, coriander, rosewood
Heart Notes: Tuberose, jasmine, rose, clove, iris, ylang-ylang, carnation, orris
Base Notes: Patchouli, vanilla, moss, amber, civet, vetiver

Giorgio Beverly Hills
Floral

Top Notes: Bergamot, mandarin, galbanum, greens, fruits

Heart Notes: Jasmine, rose, carnation, ylang-ylang, orris, lily of the valley, hyacinth
Base Notes: Sandalwood, cedarwood, musk, moss, amber

Gio (Giorgio Armani)
Floral-Fruity

Top Notes: Egyptian hyacinth, Sicilian mandarin
Heart Notes: Green jasmine, tuberose, gardenia, red rose, ylang-ylang, clove, iris balm, peach, orange blossom
Base Notes: Amber, sandalwood, vanilla

Givenchy III
Chypre-Floral

Top Notes: Aldehydes, galbanum, peach, bergamot, gardenia
Heart Notes: Jasmine, jonquil, carnation, rose, lily of the valley, orris
Base Notes: Amber, patchouli, oakmoss, myrrh, vetiver, castoreum

Gucci No.1
Floral-Aldehyde

Top Notes: Bergamot, aldehydes, lemon, hyacinth, rosewood, greens
Heart Notes: Rose carnation, jasmine, lilac, lily of the valley, heliotrope, orchid
Base Notes: Sandalwood, cedarwood, vanilla, amber, tonka bean, musk, vetiver

Gucci No.3
Chypre-Floral

Top Notes: Aldehydes, bergamot, coriander, calyx, greens

Heart Notes: Rose, jasmine, narcissus, tuberose, lily of the valley, orris

Base Notes: Amber, vetiver, patchouli, musk, moss, leather

Guess?
Oriental-Ambery

Top Notes: Mandarin orange, grapefruit, lemon, black currant bud

Heart Notes: Orange blossom, jasmine, lily of the valley, hyacinth

Base Notes: Amber, oakmoss, patchouli, orris, sandalwood, vanilla

Habanita (Molinard)
Oriental-Ambery

Top Notes: Bergamot, peach, orange blossom, raspberry

Heart Notes: Rose, jasmine, ylang-ylang, orris, heliotrope, lilac

Base Notes: Amber, oakmoss, leather, vanilla, musk, cedarwood, benzoin

Halston
Chypre-Floral

Top Notes: Melon, greens, peach, bergamot, spearmint, tagetes

Heart Notes: Jasmine, rose, marigold, cedarwood, carnation, orris, ylang-ylang

Base Notes: Vetiver, amber, patchouli, musk, sandalwood, incense, moss

Heure Exquise (Annick Goutal)
Floral

Notes: Florentine iris, Turkish rose, sandalwood

Hilfiger Athletics (Tommy Hilfiger)
Citrus
Notes: Grapefruit, bergamot, anise, greens, white sage, Utah yarrow, cottonwood, Guyana wacapua

Histoire D'Amour (Aubusson)
Chypre-Floral

Top Notes: Mandarin, bergamot, basil, osmanthus
Heart Notes: Jasmine, rose, narcissus, orange blossom, ylang-ylang, galbanum
Base Notes: Oakmoss, musk, patchouli

Hot (Bill Blass)
Oriental

Top Notes: Bergamot, rose, jasmine, lily of the valley
Heart Notes: Spices, sandalwood, cinnamon, bay leaf
Base Notes: Vanilla, amber, musk

Il Bacio
Floral-Fruity

Top Notes: Honeysuckle, rose, jasmine, freesia, orchid, lily of the valley
Heart Notes: Peach, plum, melon, passion fruit, pear, osmanthus, iris
Base Notes: Amber, sandalwood, violet, musk, cedarwood

Infini (Caron)
Floral-Aldehyde

Top Notes: Aldehydes, peach, bergamot, neroli, coriander

Heart Notes: Rose, jasmine, lily of the valley, carnation, ylang-ylang, orris
Base Notes: Sandalwood, musk, vetiver, civet, tonka bean

In Love Again (YSL)
Fruity-Floral

Top Notes: Grapes, grapefruit, brimbelle
Heart Notes: Tulip tree, grapefruit, water lily
Base Notes: Blackberry, sandalwood, mush

Ivoire de Balmain
Floral-Green

Top Notes: Jasmine, galbanum, bergamot, violet, mandarin, aldehydes
Heart Notes: Turkish rose, lily of the valley, Tuscany ylang-ylang, carnation, pepper, nutmeg, cinnamon, berry pepper
Base Notes: Vetiver, oakmoss, sandalwood, labdanum, amber, vanilla, patchouli, tonka bean

Jardins de Bagatelle (Guerlain)
Floral

Top Notes: Violet, aldehydes, lemon, bergamot
Heart Notes: Orange blossom, tuberose, magnolia, gardenia, rose, jasmine, ylang-ylang, orchid, lily of the valley, narcissus
Base Notes: Cedarwood, vetiver, patchouli, musk

Je Reviens (Worth)
Floral-Aldehyde

Top Notes: Orange blossom, aldehydes, bergamot, violet

Heart Notes: Clove, rose, jasmine, hyacinth, lilac, orris, ylang-ylang

Base Notes: Amber, incense, tonka bean, vetiver, musk, moss, sandalwood

Jean-Paul Gaultier
Floral-Fruity

Top Notes: Bulgarian rose, Chinese star anise, Tunisian orange blossom, Italian tangerine

Heart Notes: Indian ginger, orchid, Florentine Iris, ylang-ylang, rose, orange blossom

Base Notes: Reunion Island vanilla, amber, musk

Jessica McClintock
Floral-Green

Top Notes: Black currant bud, bergamot, basil, ylang-ylang

Heart Notes: Rose, white jasmine, lily of the valley

Base Notes: Musk, woods

Jicky (Guerlain)
Fougere

Top Notes: Bergamot, lemon, mandarin

Heart Notes: Lavender, rosemary, basil, orris, tonka bean

Base Notes: Vanilla, amber, benzoin, rosewood, spices, leather

Jil Sander No.4
Floral-Oriental

Top Notes: Light rose, geranium, peach, plum, galbanum

Heart Notes: Violets, jasmine, rose, tuberose, heliotrope, ylang-ylang, carnation, tarragon, myrrh

Base Notes: Grey ambergris, moss, sandalwood, patchouli, vanilla, musk

Jolie Madame (Balmain)
Chypre-Floral

Top Notes: Gardenia, artemisia, bergamot, coriander, neroli

Heart Notes: Jasmine, tuberose, rose, jonquil, orris

Base Notes: Patchouli, oakmoss, vetiver, musk, castoreum, leather, civet

Joop! Pour Femme
Floral-Oriental

Top Notes: Neroli, bergamot
Heart Notes: Bulgarian rose, jasmine, orange blossom
Base Notes: Vanilla, sandalwood, patchouli, coumarin

Joy (Jean Patou)
Floral

Top Notes: Aldehydes, peach, greens, calyx
Heart Notes: Jasmine, Bulgarian rose, ylang-ylang, orchid, lily of the valley, orris, tuberose
Base Notes: Sandalwood, musk, civet

K de Krizia
Floral

Top Notes: Aldehydes, peach, hyacinth, bergamot, neroli
Heart Notes: Jasmine, narcissus, orange blossom, rose, carnation, orchid, lily of the valley, orris
Base Notes: Sandalwood, vetiver, musk, amber, moss, civet, vanilla, styrax, leather

KL (Karl Lagerfeld)
Oriental-Spicy

Top Notes: Orange, bergamot, spices
Heart Notes: Clove, cinnamon, pimento, rose, jasmine, ylang-ylang, orchid
Base Notes: Amber, myrrh, vanilla, patchouli, labdanum, olibanum, benzoin, civet, styrax

Knowing (Estee Lauder)
Chypre-Floral

Top Notes: Greens, coriander, orange, aldehydes
Heart Notes: Rose, jasmine, lily of the valley, cedarwood, cardamom
Base Notes: Amber, sandalwood, patchouli, spices, vetiver, orris, oakmoss

L'Air du Temps (Nina Ricci)
Floral

Top Notes: Bergamot, peach, rosewood, neroli
Heart Notes: Gardenia, carnation, jasmine, May rose, ylang-ylang, orchid, lily, clove, orris
Base Notes: Ambergris, musk, vetiver, benzoin, cedarwood, moss, sandalwood, spices

L'Arte de Gucci
Chypre-Floral

Top Notes: Bergamot, fruits, coriander, aldehydes, greens
Heart Notes: Rose, jasmine, lily of the valley, mimosa, tuberose, narcissus, geranium, orris
Base Notes: Amber, musk, oakmoss, patchouli, leather, vetiver

L'Heure Bleue (Guerlain)
Floral-Ambery

Top Notes: Bergamot, lemon, coriander, neroli
Heart Notes: Bulgarian rose, iris, heliotrope, jasmine, ylang-ylang, orchid
Base Notes: Vanilla, sandalwood, musk, vetiver, benzoin

L'Insolent (Charles Jourdan)
Floral

Top Notes: Bergamot, mandarin, cassie, peach, pineapple
Heart Notes: Tuberose, jasmine, orange blossom, lily of the valley, coriander, carnation, rosewood
Base Notes: Amber, oakmoss, patchouli, musk, vanilla, cedarwood

L'Interdit (Givenchy) (Discontinued)
Floral-Aldehyde

Top Notes: Aldehydes, mandarin, peach, bergamot, strawberry
Heart Notes: Jasmine, rose, jonquil, narcissus, lily of the valley, orris, ylang-ylang
Base Notes: Sandalwood, vetiver, musk, amber, cistus, benzoin, tonka bean

L'Interdit 2 (Givenchy)
La Prairie
Floral-Fruity

Top Notes: Bulgarian rose, honeysuckle, peach, tagetes, osmanthus, peony, violet leaves

Heart Notes: Orange blossom, peach, plum, tuberose, heliotrope, rose

Base Notes: Sandalwood, amber, oakmoss, patchouli, musk, cedarwood

Laguna (Salvador Dali)
Floral-Fresh

Top Notes: Moroccan lemon, Calabrian tangerine, Spanish verbana, Asian green galbanum, plum, pineapple

Heart Notes: Egyptian rose, Italian iris, lily of the valley, jasmine

Base Notes: Madagascar sandalwood, Reunion Island vanilla, amber, musk, coconut, cedarwood, patchouli

Lalique
Floral

Top Notes: Chinese gardenia, Sicilian mandarin, blackberry

Heart Notes: Grasse magnolia, Tunisian orange blossom, peony, Bulgarian rose, ylang-ylang

Base Notes: Reunion Island vanilla, Virginia cedarwood, East Indian sandalwood, Tibetan musk, Colombian amber, Yugoslavian oakmoss

Laura Ashley No.1
Floral-Fruity

Top Notes: Peach, hyacinth, bergamot, gardenia, galbanum

Heart Notes: Narcissus, rose, jasmine, orchid, clove, carnation

Base Notes: Sandalwood, musk, vanilla, cyclamen

Lauren (Ralph Lauren)
Floral-Fruity

Top Notes: Wild marigold, greens, rosewood, pineapple
Heart Notes: Bulgarian rose, lilac, violet, jasmine, lily of the valley, cyclamen
Base Notes: Cedarwood, oakmoss, sandalwood, vetiver, carnation

Le Dix (Balenciaga)
Floral-Aldehyde

Top Notes: Aldehydes, peach, lemon, bergamot, coriander
Heart Notes: Jasmine, rose, orris, lilac, lily of the valley
Base Notes: Vetiver, sandalwood, musk, amber, tonka bean, benzoin, Peru balsam

Leonard de Leonard
Floral-Green

Top Notes: Iris, aldehydes, galbanum, hyacinth, lemon, bergamot
Heart Notes: Rose, orris, lily of the valley, carnation, ylang-ylang
Base Notes: Musk, sandalwood, moss, amber, cedarwood, spices

Listen
Floral-Fruity

Top Notes: Marigold, ylang-ylang, lily of the valley, tangerine, bergamot
Heart Notes: Jasmine, rose, gardenia, violet, lilac
Base Notes: Musk, vetiver

Liu (Guerlain)

Floral-Aldehyde

Top Notes: Bergamot, neroli, aldehydes
Heart Notes: Jasmine, May rose, iris
Base Notes: Amber, vanilla, woods

Liz Claiborne
Floral-Fruity

Top Notes: Carnation, white lily, freesia, mandarin, marigold, greens, bergamot, peach
Heart Notes: Jasmine, jonquil, rose, ylang-ylang, lilac, tuberose, lily of the valley
Base Notes: Sandalwood, amber, oakmoss, musk

Lolita Lempicka
Fruity-Semioriental

Top Notes: Ivy, anise seed
Heart Notes: Violet, Iris, amarena, licorice
Base Notes: Vetiver, tonka bean, vanilla, musk, praline

Lumiere (Rochas)
Floral

Top Notes: Coriander, honeysuckle, greens, fruits, bergamot, orange blossom
Heart Notes: Magnolia, acacia, tuberose, jasmine, lily of the valley, ylang-ylang, hyacinth
Base Notes: Sandalwood, ambergris, tonka bean, cedarwood, moss, vetiver, musk

Lutece (Houbigant)
Floral-Aldehyde

Top Notes: Mandarin, aldehydes, geranium, rosewood

Heart Notes: May rose, peony, lily of the valley, cedarwood, vetiver, orris

Base Notes: Vanilla, musk, tonka bean, heliotrope, cinnamon

Ma Griffe (Carven)
Chypre-Floral

Top Notes: Gardenia, greens, galbanum, aldehydes, clary sage

Heart Notes: Jasmine, rose, sandalwood, vetiver, orris, ylang-ylang

Base Notes: Styrax, oakmoss, cinnamon, musk, benzoin, labdanum

Ma Liberte (Jean Patou)
Oriental-Spicy

Top Notes: Heliotrope, citrus

Heart Notes: Jasmine, rose, lavender, clove

Base Notes: Sandalwood, vetiver, vanilla, musk, cedarwood, patchouli, nutmeg, cinnamon

Mackie (Bob Mackie)
Floral-Oriental

Top Notes: Peach, raspberry, pineapple

Heart Notes: Jasmine, rose, jonquil, orange blossom, ylang-ylang, tuberose

Base Notes: Sandalwood, vetiver, patchouli, amber, musk

Madame Rochas
Floral-Aldehyde

Top Notes: Hyacinth, neroli, aldehydes, greens, lemon

Heart Notes: Bulgarian rose, jasmine, iris, lily of the valley, violet, orris, narcissus, tuberose
Base Notes: Amber, cedarwood, sandalwood, moss, vetiver, musk, tonka bean

Mademoiselle Ricci
Floral-Ambery

Top Notes: Galbanum
Heart Notes: Kazanlick rose, Florentine iris, royal lily, honeysuckle
Base Notes: Patchouli, sandalwood

Magie Noire (Lancome)
Oriental-Ambery Spicy

Top Notes: Hyacinth, cassie, bergamot, raspberry, galbanum
Heart Notes: Jasmine, ylang-ylang, Bulgarian rose, lily of the valley, narcissus, honey, tuberose, orris
Base Notes: Spices, sandalwood, ambergris, cedarwood, patchouli, oakmoss, musk, civet

Maroussia (Slava Zaitsev)
Floral-Oriental

Top Notes: Ylang-Ylang, narcissus, black currant bud
Heart Notes: Rose, jasmine, orange blossom, lily of the valley
Base Notes: Amber, musk, vanilla, sandalwood

Michelle (Balenciaga)
Floral

Top Notes: Aldehydes, peach, coconut, greens, gardenia

Heart Notes: Jasmine, ylang-ylang, rose, iris, tuberose, carnation, orchid

Base Notes: Musk, vetiver, vanilla, benzoin, moss, sandalwood

Miss Balmain
Chypre-Floral

Top Notes: Gardenia, coriander, citrus, aldehydes

Heart Notes: Jasmine, rose, carnation, narcissus, orris, jonquil

Base Notes: Castoreum, patchouli, oakmoss, leather, vetiver, amber

Miss Dior (Christian Dior)
Chypre-Fruity

Top Notes: Bergamot, aldehydes, clary sage, gardenia, galbanum

Heart Notes: Rose, jasmine, lily of the valley, carnation, orris

Base Notes: Patchouli, oakmoss, amber, vetiver, sandalwood, leather

Mitsouko (Guerlain)
Chypre-Fruity

Top Notes: Peach, bergamot, hesperides
Heart Notes: Lilac, rose, jasmine, ylang-ylang
Base Notes: Vetiver, amber, oakmoss, cinnamon, spices

Molinard de Molinard
Floral-Fruity

Top Notes: Fruits, citrus, black currant bud, greens

Heart Notes: Bulgarian rose, Grasse jasmine, narcissus, ylang-ylang

Base Notes: Amber, Reunion Island vetiver, incense

Montana (Claude Montana)
Chypre-Floral

Top Notes: Peach, plum, pepper, cassie, cardamom, greens

Heart Notes: Ginger, tuberose, rose, carnation, sandalwood, jasmine, ylang-ylang

Base Notes: Patchouli, amber, castoreum, vetiver, civet, musk, olibanum

Moods (Krizia)
Floral-Fresh

Top Notes: Greens, bergamot, lemon, fruits

Heart Notes: Lily of the valley, cyclamen, orchid, jasmine, rose, carnation, orris

Base Notes: Cedarwood, musk

Moschino
Floral-Oriental

Top Notes: Coriander, galbanum, origan

Heart Notes: Ylang-Ylang, gardenia, rose, carnation, patchouli, pepper, nutmeg, sandalwood

Base Notes: Musk, vanilla, amber

Must de Cartier
Oriental-Ambery

Top Notes: Bergamot, tangerine, lemon, aldehydes, peach, rosewood

Heart Notes: Jasmine, leather, carnation, ylang-ylang, orris, orchid

Base Notes: Musk, amber

My Sin (Lanvin)
Floral-Aldehyde

Top Notes: Aldehydes, bergamot, lemon, clary sage, neroli

Heart Notes: Ylang-ylang, jasmine, rose, clove, orris, lily of the valley, jonquil, lilac

Base Notes: Vanilla, vetiver, musk, cedarwood, sandalwood, tolu, styrax, civet

Mystere (Rochas)
Chypre-Floral

Top Notes: Galbanum, cascarilla, coriander, hyacinth

Heart Notes: Violet, narcissus, May rose, jasmine, tuberose, lily of the valley, carnation, ylang-ylang, orris

Base Notes: Cypress, oakmoss, cedarwood, musk, civet, patchouli, styrax

Nahema (Guerlain)
Floral-Aldehyde

Top Notes: Peach, bergamot, greens, aldehydes

Heart Notes: Rose, hyacinth, Bulgarian rose, ylang-ylang, jasmine, lilac, lily of the valley

Base Notes: Passion fruit, Peru balsam, benzoin, vanilla, vetiver, sandalwood

Narcisse Noir (Caron)
Floral-Oriental

Top Notes: Orange blossom, bergamot, petitgrain, lemon
Heart Notes: Rose, jasmine, jonquil
Base Notes: Persian black narcissus, musk, civet, sandalwood

Nicole Miller
Aura-Floral, vanilla

Top Notes: Mandarin, cyclamen, freesia, ylang-ylang, peach
Heart Notes: Jasmine, tuberose, rose absolute, lilac, clove, orange blossom, heliotrope
Base Notes: Sandalwood, vanilla, amber, musk, tonka bean, opopanax

Niki de Saint Phalle
Chypre-Floral

Top Notes: Greens, peach, bergamot, spearmint, artemisia
Heart Notes: Jasmine, carnation, rose, ylang-ylang, cedarwood, orris, patchouli
Base Notes: Oakmoss, sandalwood, leather, musk, amber

Nina (Nina Ricci)
Floral

Top Notes: Bergamot, greens, basil, lemon, peach, cassie, tagetes, aldehydes
Heart Notes: Jasmine, rose, orange blossom, marigold, mimosa, violet, ylang-ylang, bay leaf, orris
Base Notes: Vetiver, sandalwood, patchouli, moss, civet, musk

Nocturnes (Caron)
Floral Aldehyde

Top Notes: Aldehydes, bergamot, mandarin, greens
Heart Notes: Rose, jasmine, ylang-ylang, tuberose, stephanotis, lily of the valley, orris, cyclamen
Base Notes: Vanilla, amber, musk, sandalwood, vetiver, benzoin

Noir for Women (Pascal Morabito)
Floral

Top Notes: Black currant bud, mandarin
Heart Notes: Jasmine
Base Notes: Iris

Norell (Revlon)
Floral

Top Notes: Greens, reseda, galbanum
Heart Notes: Carnation, hyacinth, rose, jasmine
Base Notes: Musk, iris, sandalwood

Nude (Bill-Blass)
Floral-Aldehyde

Top Notes: Aldehydes, rosem galbanum, narcissus
Heart Notes: Jasmine, ylang-ylang, mosses
Base Notes: Musk, sandalwood, vetiver, orris

Nuit de Noel (Caron)
Oriental

Top Notes: Citrus
Heart Notes: Rose, orris, jasmine, ylang-ylang
Base Notes: Sandalwood, vanilla, oakmoss

Obsession (Calvin Klein)
Oriental-Ambery

Top Notes: Mandarin, bergamot, peach, lemon, orange blossom, greens
Heart Notes: Coriander, tagetes, armoise, jasmine, rose, cedarwood, sandalwood
Base Notes: Vanilla, amber, oakmoss, musk, civet

Oh La La! (Azzaro)
Oriental

Top Notes: Raspberry, peach, mandarin, bergamot, fig leaves, muscat grape
Heart Notes: Yellow rose, jasmine, narcissus, ylang-ylang, orange blossom, osmanthus
Base Notes: Cinnamon, sandalwood, amber, vanilla, patchouli, tonka bean

Ombre Rose (Jean-Charles Brousseau)
Floral-Aldehyde

Top Notes: Aldehydes, peach, rosewood, geranium
Heart Notes: Lily of the valley, ylang-ylang, rose, orris, sandalwood, cedarwood, vetiver
Base Notes: Vanilla, honey, iris, musk, cinnamon, tonka bean, heliotrope

1000 (Jean Patou)
Floral

Top Notes: Greens, bergamot, anjelica, coriander, tarragon
Heart Notes: Chinese osmanthus, jasmine, rose, lily of the valley, violet, iris, geranium
Base Notes: Vetiver, patchouli, moss, sandalwood, amber, musk, civet

O Oui (Lancome)
Floral

Top Notes: Clementine, bergamot, nectarine, freesia, water hyacinth

Heart Notes: Water lily, honeysuckle

Base Notes: Frosted musk, soft woods

Opium (YSL)
Oriental-Spicy

Top Notes: Plum, hesperides, clove, coriander, pepper, bay leaf

Heart Notes: Jasmine, rose, carnation, lily of the valley, cinnamon, peach, orris

Base Notes: Sandalwood, vetiver, myrrh, opopanax, labdanum, benzoin, benjamin, castoreum, amber, incense, musk, patchouli, tolu

Oscar de la Renta
Floral-Ambery

Top Notes: Orange blossom, coriander, cascarilla, basil, peach, gardenia

Heart Notes: Jasmine, tuberose, ylang-ylang, May rose, lavender, orchid

Base Notes: Clove, sandalwood, amber, myrrh, lavender, patchouli, opopanax

Paloma Picasso
Chypre-Floral

Top Notes: Bergamot, neroli, lemon, ambrette

Heart Notes: Jasmine, Bulgarian rose, ylang-ylang, coriander, clove

Base Notes: Patchouli, vetiver, sandalwood, oakmoss, moss, amber

Panthere (Cartier)
Floral-Ambery

Top Notes: Ginger, pepper
Heart Notes: Jasmine, narcissus, rose, tuberose, gardenia, heliotrope, carnation, ylang-ylang
Base Notes: Musk, sandalwood, patchouli, amber, oakmoss, cedarwood, vanilla, tonka bean

Paradox (Jacomo)
Floral-Oriental

Top Notes: Italian tangerine, black currant bud, melon
Heart Notes: Ylang-ylang, jasmine, cedarwood
Base Notes: Haitian vetiver, sandalwood, vanilla, caramel

Parfum D'Hermes
Semi-Oriental

Top Notes: Aldehydes, bergamot, galbanum, hyacinth
Heart Notes: Egyptian jasmine, Florentine iris, Nossi-be ylang-ylang, Bulgarian rose, labdanum
Base Notes: Cedarwood, vetiver, sandalwood, amber, spices, incense, myrrh, vanilla

Parfum Sacre (Caron)
Oriental-Spicy

Top Notes: Pepper, cinnamon, coriander, clove
Heart Notes: Rose, jasmine, orange blossom, mimosa
Base Notes: Myrrh, musk, amber, vanilla

Paris (YSL)
Floral

Top Notes: Rose petals, orange blossom, mimosa, cassia, hawthorn, nasturtium, bergamot, greens, hyacinth

Heart Notes: Rose, violet leaves, jasmine, orris, ylang-ylang, lily of the valley, lily, linden blossom

Base Notes: Sandalwood, amber, musk, moss, iris, cedarwood, heliotrope

Parure (Guerlain)
Chypre-Floral

Top Notes: Plum, bergamot, fruits, hesperides, greens

Heart Notes: Rose, lilac, jasmine, lily of the valley, jonquil, narcissus, orris

Base Notes: Oakmoss, patchouli, spices, amber, leather

Passion (Annick Goutal)
Floral

Notes: Jasmine, tuberose, vanilla

Pavlova
Floral

Top Notes: Hyacinth, bergamot, galbanum, black currant bud

Heart Notes: Rose, jasmine, tuberose, orchid, narcissus, orris

Base Notes: Sandalwood, musk, amber, cedarwood, benzoin, moss

Petite Cherie (Annick Goutal)
Fruity

Notes: Peach, pear, grass, vanilla, rose
Pheromone (Marilyn Miglin)
Green

Top Notes: Greens, spices
Heart Notes: Florals, jasmine
Base Notes: Woods, bark, seeds, wine resins, wild grasses

Poison (Christian Dior)
Floral-Ambery

Top Notes: Coriander, plum, pimento, anise, rosewood
Heart Notes: Rose, tuberose, orange blossom, honey, cinnamon, wild berries, cistus, labdanum, carnation, jasmine
Base Notes: Sandalwood, cedarwood, vetiver, musk, vanilla, heliotrope, opopanax

Prelude (Balenciaga)
Oriental-Spicy

Top Notes: Aldehydes, bergamot, orange, pimento
Heart Notes: Carnation, jasmine, rose, ylang-ylang, orchid, cinnamon
Base Notes: Amber, vanilla, patchouli, civet, benzoin, tolu, olibanum

Private Collection (Estee Lauder)
Chypre-Green

Top Notes: Greens, hyacinth, citrus
Heart Notes: Jasmine, narcissus, rose, pine, reseda
Base Notes: Oakmoss, cedarwood, amber, musk

Quadrille (Balenciaga)
Floral

Top Notes: Plum, peach, lemon
Heart Notes: Jasmine, clove, cardamom
Base Notes: Amber, musk

Quartz (Molyneux)

Floral-Fruity

Top Notes: Peach, hyacinth, cassie
Heart Notes: Jasmine, rose, carnation, orris, melon
Base Notes: Sandalwood, musk, amber, moss, benzoin, cedarwood

Quelques Fleurs L'Original (Houbigant)
Floral

Top Notes: Greens, bergamot, orange blossom, lemon, tarragon
Heart Notes: Rose, jasmine, tuberose, lily of the valley, ylang-ylang, carnation, helitrope, orchid, orris
Base Notes: Sandalwood, oakmoss, amber, musk, tonka bean, civet

Raffinee (Houbigant)
Floral-Oriental

Top Notes: Orange blossom, bergamot, plum, clary sage
Heart Notes: Osmanthus, jasmine, tuberose, ylang-ylang, rose, carnation, orchid
Base Notes: Sandalwood, spices, vetiver, cinnamon, vanilla, musk

Realities (Liz Claiborne)
Floral-Oriental

Top Notes: Bergamot, chamomile, sage, osmanthus
Heart Notes: Bulgarian rose, jasmine, white lily, carnation, freesia
Base Notes: Vanilla, amber, sandalwood, peach

Realm (Erox)
Oriental

Top Notes: Sicilian mandarin, Italian cassia, Egyptian tagetes

Heart Notes: Water lily, peony

Base Notes: Honey, vanilla

Red (Giorgio Beverly Hills)
Floral-Aldehyde

Top Notes: Osmanthus, ylang-ylang, orange blossom, peach, bergamot, spices, cassie, tagetes, hyacinth, cardamom, aldehydes

Heart Notes: Jasmine, carnation, Bulgarian rose, marigold, May rose, gardenia, tuberose, orris, ily of the valley

Base Notes: Amber, musk, patchouli, sandalwood, oakmoss, vetiver, tonka bean, cedarwood, vanilla, labdanum

Red Door (Elizabeth Arden)
Floral-Ambery

Top Notes: Rose, ylang-ylang, peach, plum

Heart Notes: Winter Oriental orchid, jasmine, lily of the valley, Moroccan orange blossom, forest lilies, wild violets, freesia, tuberose, rose

Base Notes: Vetiver, honey, cedarwood, sandalwood, amber, heliotrope, musk, benzoin

Rive Gauche (YSL)
Floral-Aldehyde

Top Notes: Aldehydes, bergamot, greens, peach

Heart Notes: Magnolia, jasmine, gardenia, geranium, iris, ylang-ylang, rose, lily of the valley

Base Notes: Mysore sandalwood, Haitian vetiver, tonka bean, musk, moss, amber

Roma (Laura Biagiotti)
Oriental-Ambery

Top Notes: Sicilian bergamot, black currant bud, mint
Heart Notes: Rose, jasmine, lily of the valley, carnation
Base Notes: Civet, castor, Singapore patchouli, Yugoslavian oakmoss, balsano, myrrh, Siamese ambergris, vanilla

Romeo Gigli
Floral-Fruity

Top Notes: Sicilian lime, bergamot, mandarin, mango, black currant bud
Heart Notes: Orange blossom, rose, lily of the valley, jasmine, white carnation
Base Notes: Incense, iris, sandalwood

Rose Cardin (Pierre Cardin)
FLoral-Oriental

Top Notes: Moroccan tarragon, clove, nutmeg, coriander, rosewood
Heart Notes: Spicy rose, jasmine, peach, apricot, iris, lily of the valley, ylang-ylang, carnation
Base Notes: Honey, sandalwood, vanilla, amber, patchouli, musk

Royal Secret (Germaine Monteil)
Oriental

Top Notes: Citrus, African orange
Heart Notes: Bulgarian rose, jasmine
Base Notes: Sandalwood, musk, myrrh

Rumba (Balenciaga)
Chypre-Floral

Top Notes: Mirabelle plum, peach, orange blossom, raspberry

Heart Notes: Magnolia, tuberose, orchid, gardenia, jasmine, carnation, heliotrope, honey, lily of the valley

Base Notes: Amber, oakmoss, vanilla, sandalwood, cedarwood, tonka bean, musk, styrax

Safari (Ralph Lauren)
Floral-Green

Top Notes: Tagetes, orange, hyacinth, black currant bud, jonquil, mandarin, galbanum

Heart Notes: Italian jasmine, orange blossom, orris, genet, May rose, narcissus

Base Notes: Sandalwood, cedarwood, vetiver, patchouli, amber

Salvador Dali
Floral-Aldehyde

Top Notes: Aldehydes, mandarin, bergamot, basil, greens

Heart Notes: Jasmine, lily of the valley, tuberose, rose, narcissus, orris

Base Notes: Cedarwood, amber, vanilla, sandalwood, musk, benzoin

Salvatore Ferragamo

Top Notes: Anise absolute, neroli absolute, cassis absolute, green leaves

Heart Notes: Iris, rose, peony, nutmeg, pepper, lily of the valley

Base Notes: Raspberry, exotic woods, sweet almond, musk

Samsara (Guerlain)
Floral-Oriental

Top Notes: Bergamot, peach, lemon, greens
Heart Notes: Jasmine, orris, ylang-ylang, rose, narcissus, santal
Base Notes: Amber, vanilla, sandalwood, tonka bean, musk

Scaasi (Arnold Scaasi)
Floral

Top Notes: Apricot, mandarin, rose, coriander, orange blossom, bergamot, greens
Heart Notes: Narcissus, tuberose, jasmine, carnation, violet, rose, ylang-ylang, gardenia
Base Notes: Amber, oakmoss, sandalwood, vetiver, musk, vanilla, civet

Scherrer 2 (Jean-Louis Scherrer)
Floral-Aldehyde

Top Notes: Aldehydes, peach, mandarin, pineapple, anise, greens, bergamot
Heart Notes: Rose, lily of the valley, jasmine, orris, lily, honey, tuberose
Base Notes: Vanilla, sandalwood, amber, heliotrope, musk, benzoin

Senso (Ungaro)
Floral-Fruity

Top Notes: Grapefruit, bergamot
Heart Notes: Orange blossom, rose, jasmine
Base Notes: Peppery carnation, sweet rose, jasmine

Shalimar (Guerlain)
Oriental

Top Notes: Bergamot, lemon, hesperides
Heart Notes: Jasmine, iris, rose, patchouli, vetiver
Base Notes: Vanilla, incense, opopanax, sandalwood, musk, civet, ambergris, leather

Smalto Donna (Francesco Smalto)
Floral-Fruity

Top Notes: Living blue iris, Sicilian mandarin, living pear, tagetes
Heart Notes: Tuberose, clove, orange blossom, ylang-ylang
Base Notes: Indian sandalwood, opopanax, honey

Society by Burberrys
Floral

Top Notes: Black currant bud, tuberose, orange blossom, osmanthus, bergamot, hyacinth, greens
Heart Notes: Jasmine, mimosa, iris, ylang-ylang, gardenia, rose, orchid, lily of the valley
Base Notes: Patchouli, oakmoss, myrrh, frankincense, cedarwood, amber, musk, vanilla

Sonia Rykiel
Semi-Oriental

Top Notes: Mandarin, ylang-ylang, Hinoki wood, passion flower
Heart Notes: Jasmine, May rose, lily of the valley, iris, sandalwood, patchouli
Base Notes: Vanilla, amber, tonka bean, benzoin

Spellbound (Estee Lauder)
Floral-Ambery

Top Notes: Fruits, rosewood, coriander, orange blossom, pimento

Heart Notes: Rose, jasmine, tuberose, carnation, lily of the valley, carnation, heliotrope

Base Notes: Vanilla, amber, cedarwood, benzoin, musk, civet, opopanax

S.T. Dupont Pour Femme
Floral

Top Notes: Blackcurrent leaf, mandarin, melon, passionfruit

Heart Notes: Cyclamen, jasmine, ylang-ylang, gardenia, magnolia, rose

Base Notes: Rosewood, patchouli, oak moss, amber

Sublime (Jean Patou)
Floral-Oriental

Notes: flowers, jasmine, rose, amber, musk

Sunflowers (Elizabeth Arden)
Floral-Fruity

Top Notes: Bergamot, melon, peach
Heart Notes: Jasmine, cyclamen, tea rose, osmanthus
Base Notes: Sandalwood, musk, moss

Sung (Alfred Sung)
Floral-Green

Top Notes: Orange, ylang-ylang, mandarin, bergamot, galbanum, lemon, hyacinth

Heart Notes: Osmanthus, genet, jasmine, iris, lily of the valley

Base Notes: Vanilla, orange blossom, sandalwood, ambrette, vetiver

Sunset Boulevard (Gale Hayman)

Top Notes: Ylang-ylang, green ivy, Italian lemon, waterlilies, bergamot
Heart Notes: Jasmin, orange flower, cyclamen flower, lily of the valley
Base Notes: Musk, Haitian vetiver, Mousse de Chine, amber, sandalwood

Tamango (Leonard)
Floral-Aldehyde

Top Notes: Aldehydes, hyacinth, iris, wild orchid
Heart Notes: Rose, lily of the valley, jasmine
Base Notes: Sandalwood, oakmoss, vetiver, musk

Tatiana
Floral

Top Notes: Orange blossom, bergamot, greens
Heart Notes: Jasmine, jonquil, tuberose, narcissus, rose
Base Notes: Sandalwood, musk, civet

Teatro Alla Scala (Krizia)
Oriental-Spicy

Top Notes: Coriander, bergamot, aldehydes, fruits
Heart Notes: Rose, jasmine, ylang-ylang, carnation, tuberose, geranium, orris, beeswax
Base Notes: Patchouli, vetiver, civet, moss, musk, cistus, benzoin

Tendre Poison (Christian Dior)
Floral-Fresh

Top Notes: Galbanum, mandarin
Heart Notes: Freesia, orange, honey
Base Notes: Vanilla, sandalwood

Theorema (Fendi)
Oriental

Top Notes: California tangelos, Thai Shamouti, jasmine
Heart Notes: Osmanthus, Afghan spices
Base Notes: Sandalwood, Gaiac wood, macassar, amber

360 Perry Ellis
Floral

Top Notes: Melon, tangerine, osmanthus, lily, cool blue rose
Heart Notes: Lily of the valley, lavender, water lily, sage
Base Notes: Sandalwood, vanilla, vetiver, amber, musk

Tiffany (Tiffany & Co.)
Floral-Ambery

Top Notes: Indian jasmine, Damascena rose, ylang-ylang, mandarin, orange blossom, Italian mandarin.
Heart Notes: Florentine iris, lily of the valley, black currant bud, violet leaves
Base Notes: Sandalwood, amber, vanilla, vetiver

Tocadilly (Rochas)
Fruity-Fresh

Top Notes: Cucumber, lilac
Heart Notes: Glycine, coconut
Base Notes: Sandalwood
Tresor (Lancome)
Floral Semi-Oriental

Top Notes: Rose, apricot blossom, lilac, peach
Heart Notes: Iris, heliotrope, lily of the valley, jasmine
Base Notes: Amber, sandalwood, musk, vanilla

Tribu (Benetton)
Floral-Fruity

Top Notes: African tagetes, Italian violet leaves, Belgian black currant bud, Italian mandarin
Heart Notes: Bulgarian rose, Moroccan geranium, Indonesian ylang-ylang, Egyptian chamomile, Moroccan jasmine
Base Notes: Indian sandalwood, Haitian vetiver, Yugoslavian oakmoss, Thai benzoin

Tubereuse (Annick Goutal)
Floral

Notes: Grasse tuberose

Tuscany Per Donna (Aramis/Estee Lauder)
Floral-Oriental

Top Notes: Mandarin, grapefruit, bergamot, rose, hyacinth, lily of the valley, herbs
Heart Notes: Jasmine, honeysuckle, ylang-ylang, orange blossom, violet, carnation
Base Notes: Sandalwood, vanilla, amber, musk

273 for Women (Fred Hayman)
Floral

Top Notes: Gardenia, tuberose, jasmine, peach, plum
Heart Notes: Peach, apricot, ylang-ylang, orris
Base Notes: Sandalwood, vetiver, amber, spices, cedarwood

Un Jour (Charles Jourdan)
Floral

Top Notes: Sicilian mandarin, black currant bud, peach, lemon, pineapple, greens
Heart Notes: Jasmine, white royal lily, magnolia, ylang-ylang, hyacinth
Base Notes: Virginia cedarwood, West Indian rosewood, oakmoss, musk, sandalwood

Ungaro
Oriental-Ambery

Top Notes: Neroli, jasmine, orange blossom, rose essence
Heart Notes: Turkish rose, Florentine iris
Base Notes: Tonka bean, cardamom, sandalwood, amber

V'E Versace
Chypre-Oriental

Top Notes: Bergamot, lily of the valley, Bulgarian rose, jasmine, ylang-ylang, lily
Heart Notes: Orange blossom, iris
Base Notes: Balsamic wood, incense, amber, sandalwood, oakmoss

Van Cleef & Arpels
Floral-Oriental

Top Notes: Neroli, bergamot, raspberry, galbanum
Heart Notes: Rose, jasmine, orange blossom
Base Notes: Cedarwood, vanilla, musk, tonka bean

Vanderbilt (Gloria Vanderbilt)
Floral-Oriental

Top Notes: Orange blossom, apricot, bergamot, greens, mandarin, coriander, basil
Heart Notes: Rose, jasmine, jonquil, mimosa absolute
Base Notes: Musk, amber, moss, incense, vanilla

Vendetta (Valentino)
Floral-Oriental

Top Notes: Water lily, hyacinth, orange blossom
Heart Notes: Rose, jasmine, ylang-ylang, daffodil, marigold
Base Notes: Musk, sandalwood, patchouli

Venezia (Laura Biagiotti)
Floral-Oriental

Top Notes: Wong-shi blossom, Indian mango, black currant bud, rose, geranium, prune, osmanthus
Heart Notes: Jasmine, iris, ylang-ylang, cedarwood, ambergris
Base Notes: Vanilla, civet, sandalwood, musk, tonka bean

Vent Vert (Balmain)
Green

Top Notes: Greens, orange blossom, lemon, lime, basil
Heart Notes: Rose, galbanum, lily of the valley, freesia, hyacinth, tagetes, ylang-ylang, violet
Base Notes: Oakmoss, sandalwood, sage, iris, amber, musk

Versus for Women (Versace)
Floral-Fruity

Top Notes: Raspberry, plum, black currant bud
Heart Notes: Tuberose, boronia, sandalwood
Base Notes: Iris, amber, musk

Vicky Tiel
Floral

Top Notes: Oriental mandarin, Italian bergamot, lemon, neroli, greens
Heart Notes: Jasmine, narcissus, lily of the valley, jonquil, rose, orchid, broom, ylang-ylang
Base Notes: Indian sandalwood, tuberose, camellia, oakmoss, musk, amber, heliotrope, cedarwood

Vivid (Liz Claiborne)
Floral

Top Notes: Egyptian marigold, tangerine, bergamot, violet, freesia
Heart Notes: Tiare flower, jasmine, peony, iris, lilies, Bulgarian rose
Base Notes: Sandalwood, musk, vanilla, amber

Vol De Nuit (Guerlain)
Oriental-Ambery Spicy

Top Notes: Orange, mandarin, lemon, bergamot, orange blossom
Heart Notes: Jonquil, aldehydes, galbanum
Base Notes: Vanilla, spices, oakmoss, sandalwood, orris, musk

Volupte (Oscar de la Renta)
Floral-Oriental

Top Notes: Living mimosa, living freesia, living osmanthus, tagetes, mandarin, melon

Heart Notes: Jasmine, heliotrope, ylang-ylang, carnation, lily of the valley

Base Notes: Sandalwood, amber, patchouli, incense

Votre (Charles Jourdan)
Floral

Top Notes: Hyacinth, mandarin, galbanum, cassie, spices, aldehydes

Heart Notes: French marigold, plum tree evernia, ylang-ylang, jasmine, rose, lily of the valley

Base Notes: Sandalwood, amber, cedarwood, musk, raspberry

Weil de Weil
Floral-Green

Top Notes: Tangerine, neroli, greens, galbanum, hyacinth

Heart Notes: Lily of the valley, honeysuckle, ylang-ylang, acacia farnesiana, May rose, narcissus

Base Notes: Sandalwood, vetiver, civet, musk, oakmoss

White Diamonds (Elizabeth Taylor)
Floral

Top Notes: Italian neroli, living Amazon lily, aldehydes

Heart Notes: Egyptian tuberose, Turkish rose, Italian orris, living narcissus, living jasmine

Base Notes: Italian sandalwood, patchouli, amber, oakmoss

White Linen (Estee Lauder)
Floral-Aldehyde

Top Notes: Aldehydes, peach, citrus oils
Heart Notes: Jasmine, lilac, rose, hyacinth, lily of the valley, orchid, ylang-ylang
Base Notes: Amber, cedarwood, sandalwood, honey, benzoin, tonka bean

White Shoulders
Floral

Top Notes: Neroli, tuberose, aldehydes
Heart Notes: Gardenia, jasmine, orris, lily of the valley, rose, lilac
Base Notes: Sandalwood, amber, musk, oakmoss

Wings (Giorgio Beverly Hills)
Floral-Oriental

Top Notes: Ginger lily, green osmanthus, passion flower, gardenia, marigold, blue rose
Heart Notes: Cattleya orchid, shaffali jasmine, heliotrope
Base Notes: Woods, amber, musk

With Love (Fred Hayman)
Floral-Oriental

Top Notes: Tangerine, black currant bud
Heart Notes: Jasmine, rose, tuberose, orange blossom, tagetes
Base Notes: Patchouli, sandalwood, vetiver, musk, amber, labdanum

Womanswear by Alexander Julian
Floral

Top Notes: Mandarin, black currant bud, ylang-ylang
Heart Notes: Jasmine, narcissus
Base Notes: Sandalwood, white musk, vanilla

Y (Yves Saint Laurent)
Chypre-Fruity

Top Notes: Greens, aldehydes, peach, gardenia, mirabelle, honeysuckle
Heart Notes: Bulgarian rose, jasmine, tuberose, ylang-ylang, orris, hyacinth
Base Notes: Oakmoss, amber, patchouli, sandalwood, vetiver, civet, benzoin, styrax

Youth Dew (Estee Lauder)
Oriental-Ambery Spicy

Top Notes: Orange, bergamot, peach, spices
Heart Notes: Clove, cinnamon, cassie, rose, ylang-ylang, orchid, jasmine
Base Notes: Frankincense, amber, vanilla, oakmoss, clove, musk, patchouli, vetiver, spices

Ysatis (Givenchy)
Chypre-Floral Animalic

Top Notes: Mandarin, bergamot, ylang-ylang, galbanum, orange blossom, coconut, rosewood, greens, aldehydes
Heart Notes: Rose, jasmine, polianthes, iris, tuberose, ylang-ylang, carnation, narcissus
Base Notes: Bay rum, vetiver, patchouli, oakmoss, sandalwood, clove, vanilla, amber, musk, honey, civet, castoreum.

If you are interested in making your own perfumes or scents. You should practice most of the recipes and try to make a few of the designer notes. Look for more recipes on the internet, other books or even other eBooks. I hope you enjoy making perfume at home and Thank You for your Time.

ABOUT THE AUTHOR

William Ziegler published a couple of articles on designer perfumes trends. He was seller of designer perfumes/fragrances online. William published a blog for years called "A Little Bit of Everything". He was inspired to write for other people that like to make things at home and share his knowledge of perfume, fragrances and scents. William grew up in Erie, PA, where he still resides. He cherishes his three children most of all. William Ziegler enjoys traveling, camping and gaming in his spare time.

CPSIA information can be obtained at www.ICGtesting.com
Printed in the USA
LVOW01s0151100714

393680LV00012B/174/P